THE NATURAL HEALTH BOOK

Dorothy Hall became an expert on the growing and use of herbs through the teaching of her grandfather, who was a government botanist, and of her mother who always kept a herb garden; for it was they who created and fostered her interest in herbs. Years later she was to have her own commercial herb nursery, and she began lecturing on herbal medicine. This resulted in *The Book of Herbs*, published in 1972. Then, to become a professional naturopath, she studied at colleges in Sydney, and in Germany and Switzerland in late 1973.

Now, in her busy practice, Dorothy Hall treats and advises patients for fourteen hours a day—and still remains in perfect health. She is about to found her own College of Herbal Medicine as a centre for teaching and for consultation and treatment of the ailments that natural medicine can help or prevent.

The
Natural Health
Book

Dorothy Hall

Illustrated by Richard Gregory

CHARLES SCRIBNER'S SONS
NEW YORK

First published in Australia by
Thomas Nelson (Australia) Ltd
19–39 Jeffcott Street West Melbourne 3003

1 3 5 7 9 11 13 15 17 19 I/P 20 18 16 14 12 10 8 6 4 2

Printed in Hong Kong
Library of Congress Catalog Card Number 77-74715
ISBN 0-684-15228-2

Contents

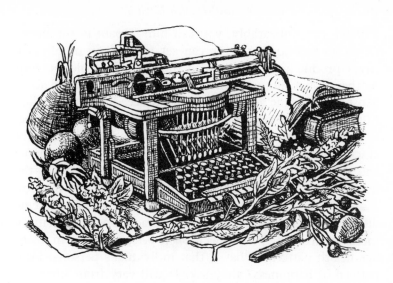

Introduction

Why do bodies degenerate and become diseased? We hear of the Hunza people who live to a tremendous age with vital health and strength; of South American communities where 120 to 130 years is the general life span; of so many other countries where the average life expectancy is only forty-five years or less, and hunger and sickness are everyday companions. Why can some people abuse their bodies with every kind of wrong food and drink and lack of exercise yet still live to a happy, healthy, ripe old age, while others can follow every new diet and every new health fad yet die of cancer or heart failure at forty? Ill-health is often the result of insufficient or incomplete knowledge of how the body works, how it removes its own garbage, and how it cleans and rebuilds itself so efficiently if given the chance. Health does not lie only with the physical body, as all of us know. When someone irritates you unbearably, you call him 'a pain in the neck'. Often an emotional trigger can set up a chain of physical stress producing a *real* pain in the neck. It could be your mother-in-law, not your sinuses, that makes your head ache! Most times, vague general ill-health proceeding if unchecked to serious illness results from *stress*. Subject a piece of steel to many pressures in many directions and it will snap or crack. Harass a human being sufficiently and his emotional and physical balance will suffer, one producing what the medical world calls mental illness and the other physical disease. And here is the first point where natural medicine differs from orthodox medicine—practitioners of natural medicine treat the patient as a *whole person*, unique in his or her health pattern. What is that individual's personal ideal pattern of happiness? they ask. It will vary from sitting in the sun all day with a bowl of fruit and Brahms on the stereo to motor-racing in dust, heat, noise and utter discomfort at 130 miles per hour. Once we understand that everyone's good health is different from everyone else's, we are well on the way to discovering our own good-health potential.

The second difference between natural and orthodox medical thought is the naturopath's belief that people react as individuals. Drugs neatly and expensively balanced to give exactly 200 mg. of this or 30 000 units of that should react beautifully with Mr Average Man—a hypothetically 'normal' person which, sadly, not a single one of us is. So natural foods and medicines are more compatible with all of us odd, different, below-par or above-average people, the body throwing away naturally whatever it cannot use, not storing it to excess in tissues and organs as it can do with many synthetic drugs and highly processed foods.

The third difference between natural and orthodox medicine is in the treatments themselves and in the correction of diet and living habits when patients come along for advice on their illnesses. Very few natural treatments are unpleasant or painful; if they are properly administered and prescribed you will find your health returning with a minimum of discomfort. I believe that if a suffering patient comes along I should not have to hurt him more to make him better, only shock him a little. It may damage his ego to be told it's time to forget the intricacies of his last golf game and the intrigues at the office and to learn a little about his body; but soon he will join in the fun of restoring and improving his own efficiency levels through common sense and understanding of the *cause* of his ill-health.

My own speciality in natural medicine is the chemical balancing of body and mind, using herbs and minerals. Of the many different natural forms of treatment, there is one or a combination of several to suit each of us: acupuncture, the ancient Chinese art of regulating and balancing physical processes now rapidly growing into world-wide acceptance; chiropractic and osteopathic treatments to adjust the skeleton, the framework of the body, so that we are functioning well mechanically, with all our nerves and blood vessels clear of harmful pressure from any out-of-place bones; massage to maintain or restore muscle function (the muscles and ligaments being the bricks and mortar that hold the bone scaffolding in place) and to improve circulation and relax tension. Many fringe areas are opening up, too: hypnotherapy to eradicate habits or circumstances that are putting stress upon the patient; hydrotheraphy, long used in the water treatments of Continental spas and resorts and now popular therapeutically for many chronic illnesses; psychic healing as practised in the Philippines—surgery without pain or instruments; colour therapy, using the electrical vibrations of different colours to produce physiological effects; and for the emotional side of us all there are yoga and meditation and new religious philosophies and creeds appearing and mushrooming as we seek peace and solutions to our problems.

This book has to do with *commonsense everyday health and happiness*, so that we can understand and correct the little things that upset us before they become big problems needing major treatment. If stinging nettles and boiled onions can help our hearts remain strong and efficient, we can then forget the strokes and the transplants and the drama attending severe heart attacks. Preventive medicine saves all of us time and effort.

If you try to run a motor-car on water instead of petrol, it doesn't really matter whether it's a Rolls or a Mini—it still won't go. If you try to fuel your body with low-grade food, it may still go—just—but it will have trouble getting up even small hills in top gear and it will cough and splutter and shudder and shake until eventually it will break down altogether, needing major repairs. Human beings can be perverse creatures who refuse to abandon habits they know are damaging to them. Those survival instincts we used to have seem to be drowned in a sea of economic necessity and time-saving! 'I haven't got time to worry about all that health thing; I've got my living to earn...'—but have you ever thought you're busily earning your *dying*, not your living?

So let's get down to some simple facts and some common-sense thinking about good health—it's easy if you know how. As with all natural processes, there are basic rules, but they're flexible. It's a matter of learning which is your particular good-health pattern.

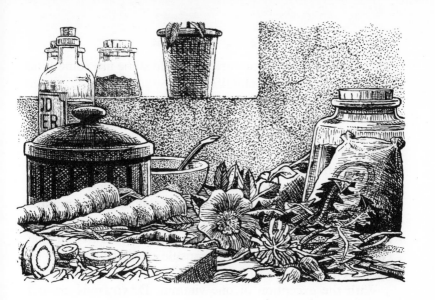

I

Vitamins

There have been so many claims made for and against vitamins that it is difficult to find a way through the piles of information available and extract the simple facts. You can read any amount of literature on vitamin E and the heart; you can espouse the cause of vitamin A as a cure-all; or you can swear by vitamin B complex as making you feel on top of the world and healthy for the first time in years: but the essential fact about vitamins is that the quantities each human body needs are enormously variable. If Mrs X next-door thrives on 5 000 units of vitamin A per day, it does not follow that Mr Y, her neighbour, will do likewise. Vitamins are perhaps the most complex agents working in our bodies: if you think the minerals are complicated you will find the vitamins are even more so. Don't be discouraged, though—persevere through this section, because without vitamins to

I

add to our mineral framework we would all be like something in a museum, without any life at all.

You can become so confused by the range and multiplicity of the vitamins on your chemist's or health store's shelves that you buy either too many or too few or the wrong ones altogether; or you can give up and say, 'For goodness' sake, I'll take a multi-vitamin capsule and be done with it!' These multi-vitamins are not the entire answer either, although they do cover a broad spectrum and supply minimal amounts of all the substances our bodies need in the way of vitamins. But each individual's need for vitamins is so different that you may take a multi-vitamin capsule every day and still be low on one or another of the group.

With the exception of one vitamin, D, vitamins are not made in the body (though the raw materials to make them should ideally be present), but must be absorbed from the food and drink we take. As the name (*vita* = life) implies, vitamins give life to the mineral and structural framework, changing and processing the raw materials into biochemical substances—that is, life-supporting and sustaining substances. Vitamins are non-mineral and are needed only in small quantities in comparison with the quantity of foodstuffs we consume in bulk each day. Most of our vitamins are manufactured by plants—which is one of the reasons why we should know as much as we can about our green growing friends in all their shapes and forms. A very good reason why we should grow as much of our foodstuffs as possible in our own backyard or area of land is that we can be sure of their comparative freedom from the toxic chemicals in sprays and preservatives. Vitamin D is the exception: as well as occurring in some herbs, it is found in animals (particularly in the livers of some fish) and is also produced by the action of sunlight on the body.

It is impossible to relate individual vitamins or the lack of them to specific diseases. Vitamins, like minerals, interact in simple combinations or in similar patterns of assimilation, and a lack of one vitamin usually means a lack of other vitamins as well. Sub-clinical symptoms of vitamin deficiency are much commoner than the acute clinical manifestations that occur with scurvy and pellagra and other serious diseases caused by extreme vitamin deficiency. You may be walking around just generally below par and in a state of chronic ill-health no matter what your pattern of living is; indeed, you may spend a great part of your life not knowing what it is to feel healthy at all if your body lacks the correct vitamin balance and is therefore unable to process your foodstuffs into fuel to power you around each day. Sub-clinical vitamin deficiency can cause pathological hunger, the type of hunger that is almost constant and is related not to appetite or to the food needs of the moment but to poor-quality food or the body's inability to process the food eaten yesterday, the day before or even last week. This kind of hunger is never satisfied, and the person so afflicted tends to eat starchy, filling foods in a vain attempt to assuage the hunger. It's the quality not the quantity of your food that counts.

Many of the isolated clinical findings about vitamins and vitamin therapy, particularly mega-vitamin therapy (that is, the prescribing of enormous doses of a particular vitamin or combination of vitamins), have given rise to quotable quotes such as, 'Vitamin A cures your skin disease', 'Vitamins of the B group help calm your nerves', and so on; and while such statements are basically true, the vitamin therapy or vitamin supplements so taken have had a naturopathic base, the revitalising of the *whole* of the human body. These vitamins and vitamin supplements are shooting you full of what you should have anyway—life-making substances; and if they are found to mitigate certain physical symptoms this is the secondary result of their initial effect on the body as a whole.

Here we are back to that basic tenet of naturopathy: 'Disease will not attack or be evident in a healthy body.'

Vitamins go a long way towards keeping each of us healthy, so of course they reduce the incidence and symptoms of a multitude of disease states.

Much scary material has been printed on the toxicity of vitamins and the terrible things they can do to you—everything from rotting your teeth to giving you diarrhoea—but excessive amounts of anything, even cold water, can have similarly harmful effects. Balance, as always, is the state we are aiming at to achieve health; so a commonsense intake of vitamins, either naturally in your home-grown food if possible, or in vitamin supplements from natural sources, will go a long way towards achieving the best possible state of health.

At present it is impossible to assess accurately anyone's exact vitamin and mineral needs (although in this age of technological inventions that time appears to be not far off). It seems to be a waste of time and effort assessing a person's needs on Monday only to find that by Friday evening those needs have changed quite considerably. A stressful day on Tuesday can throw Monday's vitamin requirements completely haywire; a sudden accident on the way home from work, a vicious onslaught of germs on Wednesday morning, or even an over-indulgence in food, drink and good company on Thursday night, can vastly change Friday's vitamin requirements.

What we must aim for is a diet that is rich in all the essential vitamin and mineral and protein foods, with the carbohydrates and fats in their right proportions. When this balance breaks down, as it will from time to time, we should then seek advice from a qualified person as to what particular vitamins or mineral supplements are needed to restore it. Many of the common diseases deplete our vitamin reserves; and of course some vitamins need to be taken each day because they cannot be stored in the body. We do not want to make our lives a misery of calorie counting, weighing ourselves each morning on the bathroom scales, and charting our vitamin and mineral intake. The state of good health we are aiming for is one in which you can eat and drink and live in such a way as to be able to *forget* about your health.

So now let's deal with each individual vitamin or member of a vitamin group and learn more about what it does once it leaves the gullet and circulates to various receiving stations in the body.

VITAMIN A

Vitamin A occurs in animals and there are sources of this vitamin in plants. It exists as vitamin A itself, a carbon, hydrogen and oxygen compound, in animals that are used for food, particularly in the livers of those animals. Plants contain carotene, which can be converted in the body to vitamin A during the digestive process. Vitamin A is present in particularly high concentrations in the livers of cod and halibut: I'll bet you all had a course of cod-liver oil at some stage or another in your early years. I remember a large greenish bottle with a white emulsified gluggy liquid in it and a picture of a North Sea fisherman in sou'wester and knee-boots on the label which sat on our kitchen dresser during the winter months when I was a child. It was my one hope after breakfast each morning that my mother would be too busy and forget my daily dose of this fishy mess. Luckily for me she very seldom did, and consequently I can count on one hand the number of colds I had as a child; and between the ages of about five and seventeen I had only one bout of influenza.

Here we have an example of vitamin A working in its role of strengthener of mucous membranes throughout the body, ensuring that these sensitive mucosal linings are strong enough to withstand attacks from passing germs. Vitamin A does not kill germs at all; it simply increases the health and resistance to germs of the soft intestinal and mucosal linings. It follows that anyone with a chronic nasal or bronchial or laryngeal infection, or any chronic excess of mucosal secretion, possibly has a deficiency of vitamin A or a defective processing mechanism for the carotene absorbed in food.

A symptom of vitamin A deficiency we all know about is night blindness, and it is the cause of many less severe eye afflictions: slight blurring of vision with no apparent organic cause, a recurrent or even constant conjunctival infection, or just an itching, burning sensation round the eyes and perhaps redness round the rims of the lids as well. Eyes are always associated with vitamin A; but remember that this is only one of the factors that control their good health.

The liver of halibut contains up to one hundred times more vitamin A than that of cod, and you may notice a variation in dose and in price of halibut-liver oil if you are able to buy this somewhat scarcer form of the vitamin. Any of the fish-liver oils contain some proportion of vitamin A, but cod and halibut have the most and are those commonly used commercially. Natural oils lose their vitamin A content rapidly as they become rancid. They are subject to chemical changes and deterioration under heat or even sunlight, so it is best to keep cooking oils and medicinal oils of any kind in the fridge or in a closed cupboard away from the light and heat. It is also best to buy cold-pressed vegetable oils—these have not been subject to any heat whatsoever and are therefore still in their pure chemical state. You will find that the best natural oil products are marketed in brown or opaque glass containers.

Vegetable sources of vitamin A are many. Apart from the green and yellow and orange vegetables there is the sweet potato, that poor relation in the vegetable bin, which is not used as much as it should be considering its rich vitamin and mineral content. Vitamin A withstands cooking well, though very high temperatures or searing can result in some loss of the vitamin content.

While we are talking about vegetables and vitamin A—one very good reason why the vegetables you grow yourself are the best is that you can avoid the use of DDT and some of the more poisonous pesticides, many of which seem to deplete the original storage of vitamin A. Diets that are low in protein do not generally use vitamin A as effectively as diets with greater protein content. Because of this, vegetarians must be very careful to supplement their vitamin A intake even more than meat-eaters do.

Anyone who has difficulty in digesting fats for any reason at all is usually low in this vitamin, and some improvement should result by simply increasing the vitamin A intake. Diabetics may have difficulty in converting carotene into vitamin A, for diabetes affects the bile, which needs to be in its healthiest and most active state for correct assimilation of this vitamin. The pure form of vitamin A may have to be added to a diabetic diet.

When we consume alcohol it carries reserves of vitamin A out of the liver and into the bloodstream, so every glass of our favourite tipple can lower our vitamin A stocks, and when we need this vitamin to repel bacterial invasion we may find there is none left. If you feel impelled to drink alcohol in any of its many forms you should be aware of what you are doing to your vitamin A reserve and take extra doses of the vitamin or foods rich in it to compensate.

Pollutant material in the atmosphere and preservative materials in foodstuffs inhibit vitamin A function and contribute to the lowering of reserve stocks in the liver. It is sadly true that almost the whole of the world's air is polluted, and an increase in our vitamin A intake is needed to counteract the life-threatening air we are obliged to breathe: this air is destructive to lung tissue which we must repair. This can become a vicious circle, in which we are continually using more vitamin A than we can naturally find to restock our supply.

If the oncoming headlights of cars blind you as you are driving at night you may have a certain degree of night blindness. If it takes you quite a few minutes to adjust from, say, a darkened theatre to the sunlight outside or from a brilliantly lit room to the darkness of the night, you may have a small degree of this limiting deficiency. Visual purple in the retina is directly related to vitamin A balance and is bleached out gradually by sunlight and light, even artificial light, during the day and regenerated in the dark while we sleep. Vitamin A controls these processes in some degree, and we only have to think of our artificially lit buildings and our lost habit of rising with the sun and going to bed at its setting to realise that this vitamin is having a harder task in civilised nations than it ever had to perform when human beings followed more natural laws. If too much artificial light and sunlight are experienced during the day there is not enough regenerative work going on in the small amount of time we spend in the dark at night to restore visual purple for the next day—yet another reason to be quite sure we have sufficient vitamin A in our diet.

This vitamin is found abundantly in cream, butter and eggs, in some margarine made from vegetable sources, as well as in the livers of fish and animals eaten as meat. Adequate sources are available, and it is up to us to ensure that what vitamin A we have is not being frittered away or is not leaking away because of alcohol consumption, pollution or any other cause: we need this good stuff ourselves!

Daylight or light of any kind, including artificial light, passes through the eyes to the pituitary gland, the vital 'control panel' of body metabolism and innumerable bodily functions. In birds and animals as well as in humans the amount of light available to the pituitary gland has been related to the functioning of many glands of the body and some of the hormones. When the days grow longer, heralding the approach of spring, birds and animals mate with a sudden surge of hormonal activity which is directly related to the pituitary function. Teenage acne is related to pituitary and hormonal function, which may have extremely erratic patterns at puberty, and vitamin A has been used with some success, in ointments and injections, to control this distressing complaint.

I have used vitamin A to treat a severe eye disease called retinitis pigmentosa; pigmentation of cells of the retina may progress until it causes a state of total blindness. The patient, having been unsuccessfully treated by her medical team, responded incredibly well to the 'bomb' of vitamin A that I gave her to arrest and then reverse the deterioration in her eyes. Her vision is improving, and I believe blindness is no longer inevitable for her. This specialised use of vitamin A is something only qualified practitioners should undertake, and I would certainly not advise you to treat yourself for such serious disorders without getting competent advice on the subject first.

In the desire to get well in a hurry, you may be tempted to overdose yourself with vitamin A: this would be extremely unwise. You would be violating the principles of natural rebuilding and restoration, and would only produce unpleasant symptoms and add to your troubles. However, even if you do overdose yourself with this vitamin for quite a long period the unpleasant symptoms will disappear very soon after you stop. Vitamin A is the 'speedy Gonzales' of the vitamin group: you react pretty fast to increasing your reserve of it, and you react even faster when that reserve becomes depleted or runs out.

Even cosmetically, vitamin A can contribute to your wellbeing: taken internally it can aid the removal of old or dead skin cells and the continued healthy growth of the remainder. Think about this vitamin and see whether your way of living has brought you enough of it or whether you could do with extra as a precaution against many forms of disease.

Foods high in vitamin A are many, but the best of them are carrots, sweet potatoes, the green leaves of beet, chicory and dandelion greens, endive, spinach (steamed), pumpkin (steamed), rockmelon, apricots (both dry and fresh), peaches, tomatoes, beef and fish liver, and eggs.

VITAMIN B GROUP

B_1—*Thiamine*

Thiamine is essential for the health of the nervous and digestive systems. It is often called the morale vitamin because lack of it results in loss of initiative, depression, failing memory, loss of concentration, rapid tiring, and poor appetite, all symptoms of a low state of mental vitality. Diets with a high proportion of refined carbohydrates tend to deplete the body's reserves of thiamine if they are not made up from other sources: thiamine is a necessity in the enzyme system whereby carbohydrates are oxidised in the tissues to give both mental and physical energy. When there is a serious deficiency of vitamin B_1 the symptoms become more acute, 'pins and needles' tingle in toes and legs, a burning sensation is often felt in the legs and feet with swelling round the ankles and accumulation of fluid there, and there may even be some signs of heart trouble. The extreme manifestation of thiamine deficiency is the crippling disease known as beri-beri, which is common among populations subsisting largely on polished rice.

Those of us who eat white bread, whether 'enriched' or otherwise, are courting disaster in the vitamin B_1 situation, for once the wheatgerm is removed from the flour in the milling process it is not possible to replace the thiamine from a synthetic source in the appropriate biodynamic form to get the same effect. You can, of course, buy wheatgerm separately: raw wheatgerm particularly is an excellent source of thiamine, for it has not been heated to stabilise it and prevent its natural deterioration. Brewers' yeast is the best natural source of thiamine in the vitamin B group, and it should be included in everyone's diet in some shape or form.

Vitamin B_1 is necessary for growth in children. Slowness of growth and weakness of the intestinal and stomach muscles can often be remedied by the addition of this vitamin to the diet. Sugar inhibits the function of thiamine and also depletes it to a certain extent, as do smoking and drinking.

Vitamin B_1 is needed especially by those of us who work very hard, for oxidation proceeds at a much faster rate with exercise, and the carbohydrates are used up more quickly.

Severe nervous disorders are often treated with thiamine as part of the therapy: these patients respond well when deficiency of the B vitamin group is part or whole of the precipitating cause.

Foods rich in thiamine are the grains and seeds, such as wheatgerm, rice bran, sunflower seed and any whole grain, brewers' yeast, nuts, legumes and potatoes; thiamine is also present in the liver of food animals. Make sure a selection of these foods is included in your diet to maintain your individual B_1 requirement. Any excess will not be stored in a harmful way in the body but will be excreted in the urine. It is best to buy the grains and seeds unbroken, in their whole state— with the husk still on them if possible. Cutting and processing, cracking and rolling, and pre-cooking or heating of any kind all reduce the amount of thiamine available from this source; but if you must cook them in some fashion, dry heat is better than cooking in water: roasting your grains fast at a medium temperature for a short period or heating them slowly for a longer time is preferable to cooking them for hours in soups or stews.

B_2—Riboflavin

Vitamin B_2 is similar in many respects to B_1 and is found in some of the same foods but more especially in dairy foods such as milk, cheese, and whey (the thin liquid left when the cream has risen to the top of the milk), in eggs, in liver, and in yeast. When our forbears milked their own cows, set their own cream each night in a big bowl on a marble slab in the pantry, churned sweet butter from some of the fat and allowed the curds to hang in muslin on their way to becoming cottage cheese; when eggs were gathered each day from hens that had foraged amongst green food and bran and pollard and such nutritious gleanings, then what healthy nerves and what vital reserves of energy, alertness, concentration and vigour those hardy ancestors would have had! How frustrating it is to us today not to be able to obtain such nutrition from simple dairy food or poultry farm sources. Do you know that up to 15 per cent of its vitamin B_2 is lost in our present-day milk when it is pasteurised and irradiated to produce vitamin D? Do you know that artificial colouring or preservative added to cheese inhibits its vitamin B_2 function? Do you know that eggs from battery-raised hens contain less than half of the riboflavin found in free-range hen eggs? It is interesting to note that these foods in their original simple, comparatively unprepared state were staple food items for country folk—and for many on the city fringes as well—two generations ago, when the mental vitality, the 'get up and go', the empire-building and the exploring and the confidence and belief in the goodness of life and the joy of living were much more in evidence.

Could our present-day miseries, our lack of confidence in the future, our resignation to the awful fate we are told awaits us, our despondency and general loss of morale, be attributed to a widespread lack of riboflavin and thiamine? It sounds far-fetched, I know, but vitamins B_1 and B_2 have been found most commonly deficient in the American diet in particular, and the symptoms of their lack follow the pattern of despondency and loss of initiative, apathy, and lack of resistance to disease under mental stress and strain. It is a sad fact that our diet has changed, in a few decades, from the simple foods enjoyed by our grandparents. It's no use trying to go back to the farm when the farm is overlaid with high-rise development and expressways; so how are we to compensate for this vital and basic lack in our food?

Only a decade or so ago wheatgerm was considered fit only

to be thrown to the pigs and fowls. Now, luckily, we know that wheatgerm is something we not only should have, but something we must have each day if our stamina and mental faculties are to continue in a state of health; and we know that a common fungus-type plant, yeast, provides an alternative if wheatgerm is not available, for it contains the B vitamin complex in balanced amounts, and is in fairly good supply in most countries. There are people who say they can't take yeast—we shall come to that later on—but for the majority of us yeast and wheatgerm can provide now what our grandparents got naturally from their simple foodstuffs simply prepared.

The most common signs of vitamin B_2 deficiency are cracks and roughness at the corners of the mouth, mouth ulcers, skin eruptions, inflamed eyelids, an intolerance to bright lights, and numbness in the legs. Sometimes vaginal inflammation is a sign of this deficiency, and usually a purplish tongue coloration is found when vitamin B_2 is seriously lacking. Sometimes you may eat exactly the right foods and still lack riboflavin because of an under-active stomach, which has insufficient hydrochloric acid and cannot assimilate the riboflavin available to it: this condition can be corrected with various natural therapeutic treatments so that the valuable vitamin can once again be absorbed. Cooking your vegetables in an alkaline solution can destroy most of the B_2 present, so don't go adding bicarbonate of soda to your beans and peas—if they are properly grown they should be green anyway.

The need for vitamin B_2 increases when the fat content of the diet is high: if you are a fish-and-chips addict you will need more B_2 than if you are a vegetarian.

Some B complex vitamins are synthesised in the intestines; so drugs that can kill natural bowel flora, such as any of the antibiotic drugs, can upset the intestinal balance and dislocate the vitamin B_2 and other vitamin B group functions to an alarming degree. If you have had any disease that caused diarrhoea lasting for longer than two or three days you most probably need a supplement of vitamins of the B group.

Red peppers—the hot variety—are extremely rich in riboflavin, as are almonds', mushrooms, the dairy products we have mentioned (in their natural state if possible), wheatgerm, yeast, lentils and beans. If you sprinkle only one dessertspoon of brewers' yeast powder every morning on your breakfast muesli, cereal, or fruit you will be ensuring that your nervous, emotional and intellectual functions are at their peak for that day.

How simple achieving natural good health can be! It's a matter of knowing what to do, then getting accustomed to the habit, then forgetting it to the extent that you do it naturally: it should be as obvious and as natural as cleaning one's teeth before bedtime to see that a certain amount of yeast and wheatgerm is in the daily diet of every man, woman and child.

B_3—*Niacin*

Niacin is the vitamin of the B group that prevents and also cures pellagra. This may not mean much to you if you don't know what pellagra is, but let me tell you that the less serious symptoms of niacin deficiency are found, like those of the other B-group vitamins, in a large proportion of our civilised populations; the extreme form of niacin deficiency is seen as pellagra in badly undernourished communities. This is a painful and destructive disease in which dementia, diarrhoea and dermatitis figure largely, and the sufferer often has a red and painful tongue, besides severe bodily weakness which can eventually cripple him. The lesser symptoms of niacin deficiency are seen in about half of us most of the time. Doesn't this combination of ailments sound like a description of someone in your own family or environment—insomnia, nausea, tender gums, indigestion with abdominal pain and loss of appetite, general irritability with anxiety in varying degrees, dizziness and fatigue, odd feelings of numbness here and there, backache, headache, some degree of depression...? Often some of these symptoms are the prelude to a nervous breakdown. So many of the people we know (and perhaps even the person we know the least, ourself!) are ready to scream, throw up their hands and go north in search of a quiet piece of land with a cow and an orchard, to get out of the rat race and search for a different system of values. It would be cheaper, instead, to take a course of natural niacin in the form of yeast tablets or natural vitamin B₃ tablets, and to discover the inner feeling of well-being that can be experienced no matter what the environment and conditions as long as one is in good health. Go bush, by all means, but try some vitamin B first, before you put the house on the market and kick the boss's teeth in!

The more white sugar and fats and protein from animal sources you eat, the smaller your reserve of niacin. Like others in the B vitamin group, this vitamin is needed to process these substances in the body. It is found in all seed foods and in animal and fish livers, in fish itself, and of course in yeast. If you are a smoker, as well as being a candidate for a nervous breakdown you're making it even harder for yourself because smoking releases adrenalin into the body (which is the reason why every cigarette you smoke can give you a little lift); but a lack of niacin upsets the balance of the adrenal gland and its secretions and your smoking may release a little energy for you but may be giving your adrenals a thump over the ear in the process. As the adrenal gland controls our 'fight or flight' mechanism—our automatic defence system if you like —you can see that any irregularity in the gland is something we can do without. If somebody came at you wielding a hatchet and yelling, your natural defence mechanism would spring almost automatically into action, and you would put your arms over your head to protect yourself, turn away and run, or perhaps you would grab the assailant. If your niacin levels were low you would be more likely to just stand there and have your head split.

When early man ate seeds and raw fish from the streams his nervous system and ability to defend himself from the slings and arrows that fortune, and other cavemen, threw at him were far superior to those of his present-day descendants. Niacin forms enzymes, those necessary and extremely complex chains of molecules that run about our bodies all day giving life and vitality and absorbing food and processing it. Niacin should really be taken together with the other B-group vitamins, but even on its own it can make you feel much more on top of your woes than underneath them.

B₅—Pantothenic Acid

Pantothenic acid is one of the more recently studied vitamins of the B group, and it appears to aid and bolster the action of other B vitamins as well as having significant properties itself. It is often called the anti-dermatitis factor and has proved beneficial for both skin and hair. Pantothenic acid has been used with success to restore prematurely greyed hair to its normal colour. If the greying is the result of a lack of this vitamin, the hair colour will return as long as irreversible change has not taken place. This vitamin can also help people whose hair is wiry and strong or very tightly curled and difficult to handle, for it tends to soften the strong-minded tresses and make them more manageable. The vitamin is water-soluble, so if you boil your seeds and grains instead of steaming them or eating them raw you will thow it out with the water: never an economical or sensible idea. Peanuts, wheatgerm, brewers' yeast, and unpolished rice, together with liver in its raw or desiccated form, are the best sources of this vitamin.

B₆—Pyridoxine

Pyridoxine, B₆, is another important member of the B vitamin complex which is found in the same foods again—wheatgerm, soya beans, peanuts, liver and yeast—and from a newer source for our B group vitamins, namely oranges and lemons and the other citrus fruits. It is soluble in water and is destroyed by prolonged sunlight and heat. It converts tryptophan to niacin, so that if you haven't enough niacin in your system, pyridoxine or vitamin B_6 will transform enzyme and protein material to provide it for you. This vitamin is another must for the fish-and-chips brigade and for people who eat foods rich in fats and carbohydrates, for it helps the body to digest fatty acids. It is of great value to the nervous system, the appetite and digestion, and greatly benefits the red blood cells and blood vessels and also the liver. It has been called the anti-convulsive vitamin and has been prescribed medically for convulsions in both children and adults. The requirement for this vitamin varies tremendously—indeed some babies are born with what appears to be a hereditary insufficiency followed by an increased demand for it. There is no absolute way yet of determining what an individual's needs for this vitamin are, but anyone with a suspected deficiency can benefit by eating the foods rich in it, or even taking supplementary doses. Experimental work is being done in the American medical world on the treatment of such serious conditions as Parkinson's disease with carefully balanced and individually adjusted injections of vitamin B_6. Vitamin therapy in massive doses or by injection is becoming quite popular with orthodox practitioners, but the patients can help themselves a great deal by including vitamin-rich foods in their everyday diet.

Folic Acid

Folic acid, often called vitamin M, is found spread generously through every green leaf that we eat raw—and preferably fresh. It is also found in beneficial quantities in mushrooms, soya beans and other beans, wheatgerm, yeast, and strawberries. Folic acid is an important factor during pregnancy—in fact it must be in its correct balance in the body before conception can take place. It is the most easily lost from foodstuffs of all the B group. If you boil or over-heat foods it will be gone in no time at all; and it is best to eat those salad greens as soon as possible after they are picked from the garden. Even mushrooms are better just washed and chopped up raw with a light dressing or added to a rice salad. You must, of course, cook dried beans after soaking them overnight in water; but remember to cook them in the water in which you have soaked them and to keep it afterwards for use in soups and stews and casseroles: some of your B vitamin constituents will still be in the water.

If you have had sulpha drugs at any time you may have experienced the depression and fatigue and general feeling of nausea that often sets in. These drugs can interfere with the helpful intestinal bacteria that make folic acid or convert foodstuffs into it. If you must take these drugs for some streptococcal infection you could take some folic acid as well, to make sure your supply is adequate and to eliminate some of the unpleasant side-effects of the drugs.

Wheatgerm and yeast contain folic acid as well; and there are two gourmet's delights amongst the foods containing a high percentage of it—oysters and salmon. That old wives' tale about oysters and increased sexual activity is not to be taken lightly: for the folic acid often helps women to conceive. It may not have been the parsley that caused the pregnancy, but the seafood cocktail!

Paraminobenzoic Acid (PABA)

A mouthful to pronounce, paraminobenzoic acid is a vitamin within a vitamin, so to speak, being a component of folic acid. It is similar to almost all of the B vitamin group in that it protects natural hair colour, preventing premature greying, is useful in skin disorders, and is thought to be useful in alleviating nervous complaints as well. It seems to protect the skin from ultraviolet damage, and one of its important uses is as a sunburn preventative. I have personal experience of the effects of over-exposure to damaging rays, not from lying on a beach too long in the summer sun but from going to sleep under an ultraviolet lamp—a lapse for which I would castigate my patients. In a spell of grey, drizzling weather in late winter I turned on my ultraviolet lamp to catch a little artificial sunshine and caught instead severe burning, with effects similar to vitiligo, a condition in which large patches of skin lose their pigment, often from ultraviolet or radiation damage. Severe electrical burns can produce the same symptoms. I had a multitude of white blotches covering neck and face and looked rather like a speckled hen for a few days until I remembered PABA and prescribed myself a series of massive doses which in a matter of days gradually and quite effectively healed the damaged skin.

Again I would advise you not to attempt to diagnose or prescribe for yourself or your family and friends. Instead, ask the advice of a qualified person who will be able to prescribe for you with knowledge and safety. This is not to say you should not take PABA in preventive and prophylactic doses as prescribed on the container—not at all. These small maintenance doses will prevent the problem occurring in the first place. Treatment of such a condition *after* it has happened is a much more serious and responsible matter, needing expert help. You can quite happily and safely take PABA on its own in early spring to prepare your body for the summer sun's onslaught if you are a beach sun-baker, but if you are taking your yeast and wheatgerm faithfully this will not be so necessary.

Choline

Choline is a favourite of mine amongst the B vitamin club because I use it so often, not isolated from the foods that contain it, but given in a form with which I am most familiar— dandelion. Every patient who comes to me with obesity problems resulting from the body's inability to process and convert fatty substances in their foodstuffs is prescribed dandelion in one way or another: either in dandelion coffee made from the root of the plant or in dandelion extract or tincture in their medicines; or I tell them to go out and pick the leaves of this free and abundant remedy for many of the ills of twentieth-century man.

Choline is one of the substances that regulates and stabilises liver function. If your liver is happy and functioning well, your built-in chemical factory is keeping the assembly lines moving to manufacture and convert every product your body needs to keep it functioning well. The proper use of cholesterol within the body is determined by the amount of choline and lecithin your liver has available to work with. If you are on a low-protein diet for any particular reason, or if you are a vegetarian who uses mainly vegetable forms of protein such as soya beans and nuts, you will have slightly less methionine (a form of protein), which needs to be present before your body can make choline. All these interdependent processes! It's no wonder your body needs sleep when you think of all the activity that goes on in every cell and organ and muscle and sinew. When enough choline is present, gained either from foodstuffs or by way of food supplements such as yeast and liver and wheatgerm, your body can manufacture lecithin, which then breaks up extra cholesterol that would perhaps otherwise form fatty deposits, clogging the walls of your arteries and heart. Cholesterol is certainly needed—indeed, it is manufactured by the body if it is not present—but unless these other factors are balanced to handle it your cholesterol is going to run amok and close up the pipes that carry your blood through your body. Then up goes your blood pressure.

You can see how involved the mechanics and biochemics are. You may not be aware of them while you are answering the telephone in your office or relaxing by the television after dinner, but your body keeps making and breaking, transforming and converting, adjusting and balancing, in true perpetual motion. What piece of machinery invented by man could continue such a complicated programme, adjusting itself as it goes without any conscious control? If you consciously control the circumstances so that they are the best possible for your body to go on with this mammoth task, then you should live a long and happy life. A few dandelion leaves picked in the park as you make your way home from work, or the dandelion leaves in the weed patch on your own footpath, can be part of your contribution to your body's equilibrium.

Soya beans and the other B-complex foods all contain choline, and so do egg yolks—and here we come across another of Nature's provisions for our health. Egg yolks contain not only a high percentage of cholesterol but the substance choline to control that cholesterol's function. I am certainly not agin' eggs as such, although, as I have mentioned before, the sadly different methods of egg production these days make one wish for the beautiful deep-pumpkin-yellow yolks and clear whites my grandmother used to poach for us— eggs laid by the hens that same morning. And, what's more, that beautiful yellow colour was not put there by synthetic dyes injected into the eggs or synthetic colouring material fed to the hens: it just happened.

We shall talk about eggs again later, in the chapter on good, bad and indifferent foods, but if you can eat egg yolks from free-range hens that have foraged amongst grass and in open air and sunlight you will be doing your whole body a good turn.

Biotin

Biotin converts unsaturated fats into body fuel. It also contains sulphur, which none of the other B vitamin group does. Sulphur is the 'kitchen broom' of the body, so biotin can claim to be a protection against infections, particularly of the streptococcal type. If you have recently had a course of antibiotics, it is possible that your biotin level is low or non-existent, since its function is inhibited by these drugs. Raw egg-white can destroy biotin; but none of us needs to live on a diet of raw egg-white, and there is nothing to stop us eating just the egg *yolk*. A deficiency of biotin can cause symptoms of anaemia, slow growth, and dermatitis on the arms and legs. The previously mentioned B-group foods contain biotin, and so do molasses, spinach, cauliflower and salmon.

Inositol

Inositol is a comparatively new discovery, classed in the B complex because it has vitamin-like activity. (We begin to wonder whether we shall ever come to the end of discovering new substances present either amongst or in relation to other substances we know already.) Its properties can be totally inhibited by the use of caffeine and the pesticide known as lindane. If you are a heavy coffee or tea drinker you will absorb caffeine from these beverages and kill off your inositol. Whatever this may mean, it would certainly not appear to be a good thing, for if a substance is found to be doing a particular job in the body it is better left there to continue doing that job. Inositol is found in the B-group foods, too.

There appears to be a connection between inositol and the elasticity of the arteries, and it also appears to regulate lecithin metabolism, associated with fat processing. Recent research in America indicates that lack of inositol can cause failure to reproduce in either male or female. Much more has yet to be learnt about inositol and its undoubtedly complicated and interrelated functioning with other substances.

B_{12}

Vitamin B_{12} is found in rubbish bins, compost heaps, rotting vegetable and animal remains, in sewage and in urine. (What peculiar places in which to find one of the most valuable vitamins of all, the growth vitamin!) Just as in other aspects of Nature, B_{12} is a substance in perfect balance between life and death: it is needed before life can begin in both humans and animals, and even in plants, and it is found to be present when humans, animals or plants return their lives to the Nature whence they came. You could call B_{12} the master catalyst, the factor that starts the process of producing life and growth as part of the cycle of living matter. You may know that vitamin B_{12} is found in liver, but the vegetarians among you may not know that it is found in really large quantities in two important plant sources—comfrey and kelp. If you include from 60 to 90 milligrams of ground kelp or a few natural kelp tablets in your diet each day, you are sure of maintaining your vitamin B_{12} levels and the growth and master control of the metabolism of nucleic acid and nucleo-proteins, substances that are part of the DNA molecule. DNA is the stuff of life itself, the difference between a living and a dead organism. You can see the importance of B_{12} in galvanising such living processes into activity. Unlike the other vitamins we are to investigate, B_{12} contains a heavy mineral, cobalt. We all know that cobalt is used by the medical profession to treat deep cancers that are either inaccessible or stubborn to other types of treatment. Possibly B_{12} contains also a cobalt 'bomb' that operates in a similar fashion within the cells, breaking down foreign or rogue cells that could cause later problems.

In civilised communities there are many reasons why B_{12} is either assimilated poorly or not assimilated at all. If you haven't enough calcium in your diet; if you haven't enough hydrochloric acid in your stomach; if your metabolic rate is too high and undigested food passes rapidly through your intestinal system; if you have abnormal bowel flora as a result of intestinal infections, prolonged use of antibiotic treatment, or parasitic bowel infestation, with chronic constipation or chronic diarrhoea: from whatever cause, it is quite likely that you are not completely or efficiently assimilating B_{12} from your diet. This is one reason why one of my favourite herbs, comfrey, is such a useful and balanced treatment for any of these problems: it not only provides calcium and the cell-proliferating substance allantoin (which facilitates reconstruction of cells and regrowth of tissue that has been seriously damaged) but it also contains the B_{12} vitamin that is manu-factured within the plant from substances drawn from the soil and the surrounding air. Comfrey not only provides healing treatment but creates circumstances in which correct functioning of the bowel is once again possible. It ensures that enough B_{12} is available to bring the body's entire metabolism back to normal.

It used to be thought that an 'intrinsic factor' was present in the gastric juices and the stomach linings of human beings and animals, which was a major factor in the correct assimilation of B_{12}. This intrinsic factor was said to be a substance present in yeast as well, so if someone had difficulty in assimilating B_{12} it was common practice to give him yeast supplements as a form of treatment. This was found to be only half a solution to the problem, for even with yeast additives such a patient might still have some difficulty with his B_{12} metabolism. It is now thought that the general biochemical programming of each individual is set to have either a greater or a lesser rate of absorption of B_{12} and a greater or lesser ability to process it. Just as you may be born with blue eyes, and no amount of taking thought can change this genetic pattern, so it may be that your B_{12} metabolism is programmed for you before birth along with your other inherited characteristics. However, even conditions predetermined in this way can be gradually restructured. You may be stuck with blue eyes and strong hair and long bones, but you may be able to change your biochemical pattern as it works in certain metabolising foodstuffs.

Such illnesses as pernicious anaemia, blood platelet disease or deficient replacement and manufacture of blood components; wasting diseases and atrophic conditions such as multiple sclerosis and muscular dystrophy; chronic and difficult metabolic patterns such as those suffered in diabetes; and deep-seated allergic reactions like coeliac disease—all these have been treated with vitamin B_{12} in doses suited to each individual. But these are matters for diagnosis and therapy rather than for home treatment, for the metabolism of the patients must be under constant surveillance.

B_{12} is found in some dairy products too—for instance,

milk and cheese—and in egg yolks and most meats. It does not need to be ingested in greater quantities than found in good foodstuffs unless there is some obvious metabolic disorder, for a healthy human being needs only a minute quantity each day. It is often referred to as the growth vitamin, and about the only time you don't need it is when you are approaching the age of puberty, and happen to have a mother who is six feet two inches tall, a father who is six feet four inches, and grandparents and uncles and aunts and cousins all well above average height. I'm not saying that tall teenagers should stop eating egg yolks or liver. Many teenagers grow so fast over a short period of time that they can tire their bodies tremendously in so doing; but they don't need some well-meaning person to suggest that a B_{12} supplement may help in overcoming the general tiredness—amounting sometimes to extreme lethargy—that can be experienced as the body works so hard at growing. If you are in any doubt as to your body's ability to stop growing it is better to obtain your energy and vitality from protein and natural carbohydrate sources that do not contain large proportions of B_{12}. Stick to balanced foodstuffs such as wheatgerm and fresh fruit and vegetables and honey and nuts.

Many of my patients have responded remarkably well to therapeutic doses of B_{12} when other treatments have failed. This vitamin is often a wonderful standby for a chronically sick person, even one who has been told that his disease is not only irreversible but is progressing fast: it will give a boost to his whole metabolism before recovery procedures are undertaken by a practitioner who does *not* admit that ill-health is unavoidable. Sometimes the use of B_{12} will return enough vitality to the sick person to enable his body to benefit quite remarkably from the recovery procedures.

VITAMIN C

If you went to school in Australia you would have been taught that Captain Cook discovered not only Australia but how to

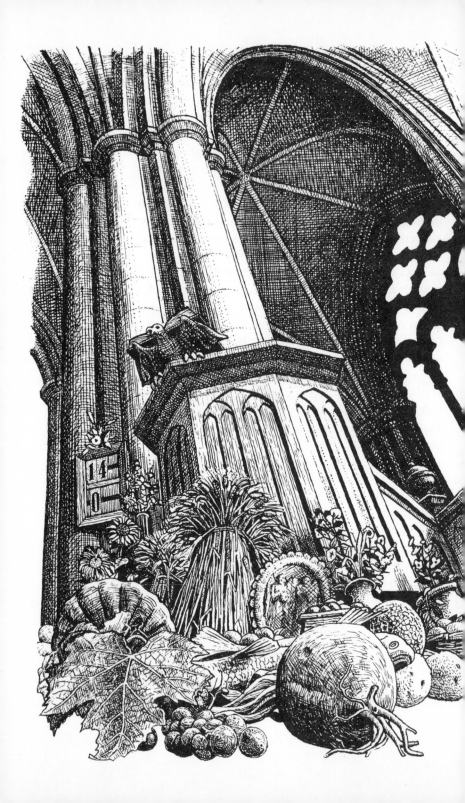

prevent scurvy occurring among his men. You may have been told, as I was, that he did this by giving the sailors lemon juice—which is not true: for he first gave his men barley sprouts and, later on, lime juice and fresh vegetables. This was sound though instinctive nutrition, for the vitamin C content of sprouted grains is very rich, and so is that of lime juice and greens. The captain's idea in giving these particular foods to his crew was that there was no deterioration on long sea voyages because the barley could be freshly sprouted every few days and the limes would keep for long periods. ɪt seems that he had been impressed with the health of native peoples as compared with that of his own men, so he copied their simple ways and reaped the benefit. He may have been the first person to set that great Australian pattern of 'give it a go'—try it out and learn from the results. It was not until the early 1900s that lemons were found by a group of food research scientists to contain vitamin C. Captain Cook's men did better with their lime juice, for limes contain more vitamin C than lemons.

Vitamin C carries hydrogen round the body, fuelling it and helping with the proper absorption of iron, that mineral so vital for oxidising or 'burning off' waste. Vitamin C is highly perishable and soon destroyed in any cooking process; and if you cut and prepare your fruit and vegetables some time before eating them, you are losing much of their vitamin C content, which leaks out through the cells of any cut surfaces. You know you shouldn't cook any vitamin-C-rich vegetables long and slowly and you know you shouldn't add bicarbonate of soda to your beans and peas to make them a lovely green colour—this destroys the vitamin C straight away (they won't need this artificial colouring if they are organically grown, anyhow).

We have all met the person who, when you say 'How are you?' answers with, 'Dreadful. I feel as if I'm falling apart.' This may be an indication of his need for more vitamin C, the cementing substance that joins the body cells one to the other. If your cells are not held strongly bonded, you may fall apart more literally than you imagine. This vitamin controls tone and resilience, and when it is absorbed in sufficient quantity to bind cells together properly, you can bounce back from either physical or emotional trauma better than you may do without it. It assists in repairing and renewing cells, and should be given in the same context as B_{12} when there has been major tissue damage, to ensure that the new cell growth at the previously damaged areas is strong and firmly held together. This is why it is prescribed for the bruising, internally or externally, that can occur after surgery or after an accident. It is not general practice in hospitals to give a massive dose of vitamin C after surgery, but this simple therapy could help in a patient's recovery to a major degree. It should also be taken before entering hospital, for several weeks if possible, so that tissues will be stronger and less subject to the shocks of anaesthetics and drugs.

The oral administration of cortisone can completely block your vitamin C absorption; so can sulpha drugs, and so can antibiotics. In major disease states for which any, and sometimes several, of these drugs may be given over a period, it would be wise to insist that the patient take a natural vitamin C supplement to try to replace that which has been lost. Smoking also throws your vitamin C metabolism sideways, and it may not be just the irritating quality of the inhaled tobacco that is tearing your throat and bronchial tree and lungs to pieces: it may also be your low vitamin C level, making it difficult to repair any damaged areas. Every cigarette you smoke removes from the metabolic processes about the amount of vitamin C you would receive from an orange: so you should eat at least two oranges for every cigarette you smoke, in order to leave vitamin C available to cope with the next cigarette. You would need a crate a day to catch up with yourself if oranges are your only source of vitamin C and you are a heavy smoker.

Spongy bleeding gums and poor teeth often indicate a

vitamin C deficiency. And if the same person has tiny capillary arteries and veins visible on the surface of the skin, reddened and discoloured because of the fragility of the blood-vessel walls, it is a stronger indication still that he is sadly lacking in vitamin C.

Another of vitamin C's jobs is to harden the dentine of our teeth. Here we find one of Nature's typical patterns where a small amount of a substance helps a condition that a large amount of the same substance destroys, for synthetic vitamin C in massive doses can contribute to breakdown of tooth enamel: anything in unbalanced *artificial* doses can contribute to breakdown of a natural process by upsetting the equation one way or another. We would be far better off with the vitamin C from rosehips or from other natural sources, for in its natural form it can only help not harm, no matter how much is taken.

There is as yet no scientific explanation for the difference in their effects between a natural and a synthetic product with the same chemical formula. The fact remains that foodstuffs containing natural, balanced compounds do not contribute to body unbalance, while foods containing synthetic compounds have been found to do so. Synthetic fluorides can inhibit the assimilation of vitamin C; and in areas where drinking water is unnaturally fluoridated by local authorities, the picture is quite different from that of areas where the drinking water is naturally high in fluorides. The natural fluorides do no harm, but synthetically fluoridated water, inhibiting the function of vitamin C, can have the opposite effect from the one intended—contributing to the breakdown instead of the hardening of tooth enamel. All we can do to counteract the harmful effects of water that has been artificially fluoridated in spite of our protests is to increase our intake of vitamin C, which detoxifies the bloodstream and carries fluorides out of the system in the urine.

You may be saying, 'I want to be one of those people who have enough vitamin C to beat any disease state, but how can I do this naturally when this vitamin is so perishable and so easily lost?' The answer, in one word, is rosehips. Rosehips are the orange hips or pods of the common dogrose, *Rosa canina*, which is found growing wild all over railway embankments and roadsides in Europe and North America. In parts of Australia it is happily beginning to be found in patches here and there by the roadsides. These bright little orange-red acorn-shaped hips are a different animal altogether from the yellow-orange, round, sad-looking ones on garden roses. Don't confuse the two—the hips of the wild rose are the only ones worth using. Rosehips contain between 500 and 6000 milligrams of vitamin C for every hundred grams of their weight. If you have a cup of rosehip tea each day, there is your vitamin C from a natural source in a pleasant form without any side-effects. Use it not only when you are sick but in its preventive role when you are feeling comparatively healthy. You can add a little honey or lemon juice to your cup of ruby-red liquid, and what a pleasant change it is from the usual mid-morning cup of tea!

Green and red peppers are extremely good sources of vitamin C and easy to grow in your garden; brussels sprouts are another source, and it may surprise you to know that there is more vitamin C in one guava than there is in three oranges. There's that vitamin C-iron balance in parsley; then there is the fruit of the acerola, a type of cherry and the second highest source (after rosehips) of vitamin C in a natural form. Blackcurrant juice we all know of as a good source of vitamin C, particularly for a young child who has a cold or an infectious disease condition; blackcurrant juice is pleasant to take and has a cooling effect on the body. Amongst the vegetable herbs we find watercress and dandelion greens, both very high in this vitamin and both freely available naturally. Lemon juice, orange juice, and grapefruit juice we all know about: so many diets, to keep us healthy, start with a glass of orange or lemon or grapefruit juice first thing in the morning to ensure that our vitamin C is present for the rest of the day. Even sweet potato contains vitamin C, and you will find that all the berry fruits and all the green vegetables contain it in high proportions. Tropical fruits such as rockmelons and mangoes and papaws are rich in this vitamin, and orange peel is nearly three times richer in it than the juice of the orange itself. Fresh red cabbage is a good source, as are kale and mustard greens, also dock, that common weed growing along our highways and ditches whose leaves could be added to our green salad bowl at no cost whatever. Strawberries contain vitamin C in significant amounts—indeed, any fresh fruit or vegetable you can eat will help along your vitamin C quota. Sometimes C is called the 'anti-stress' vitamin: it follows that we all need more of it now than we did one or two generations ago. It is stored in its greatest concentration in the adrenal gland, which controls our kidney function as well as our 'fight-back' mechanism in disease and our vitality in health. If you want to have that vital, alive look that is so rare in our busy cities, try vitamin C to help you acquire it.

It is not possible to get too much vitamin C, for any excess is excreted in the urine; but some people, including myself, do not appear to have a good dietary tolerance to high doses of this vitamin. I have often wondered why this is so, and recent reading on research done in America seems to give the answer: for there is some evidence that if sufficient other vitamins are present in the body vitamin C can be produced by the human organism. How Nature provides! We can eat a lot of useless bulk-type foods that contribute little dietetically, and Nature, to preserve our sad and inadequate species, allows us to change or mutate. This little ray of sunshine from human research seems to indicate that humankind will continue adapting itself to its environment. I firmly believe that no disaster, either man-made or natural, will wipe our species out: man has the adaptability of a chameleon. While this is not an excuse for going lightly on your vitamin C, it is a hope for the future of our species that we may need less vitamin C some hundred generations from now, being able to manufacture our own.

Those people who have an intolerance to natural vitamin C, such as occurs in rosehips and orange juice, may react in that way because they have sufficient of the other vitamins in their natural diet to enable their bodies to manufacture some vitamin C. This could be Nature's way of telling us that we do not need any extra.

We usually think of vitamin A in connection with eyesight and vision, and vitamin C relates to the eyes as well, not in their functional but in their structural sense. There is little or no vitamin C to be found in an unhealthy eye: the eyes of people suffering from cataracts have none. Vitamin C has therefore been used therapeutically in the treatment of cataract, and with marked success. But don't attempt to diagnose or treat your own condition: ask the advice of those who are trained in this field.

Nature also knows best in providing vitamin C in enormous quantities in mother's milk. No one needs protection from the assaults of this world more than a newborn child, and this, for me, settles the argument entirely as to whether or not a child should be breast-fed. If his mother's milk is available that is what he should have: for its vitamin C content alone, it is the obvious food in the required proportions to safeguard the child in its vulnerable first few months of life. The vitamin C in the milk also activates enzyme patterns in the body, and the child has therefore more 'life' and vitality as the enzyme-trains go into their act of using the food and breaking it down into other components ready to become available to the cells.

New sources of vitamin C are being discovered in so-called backward countries: an acid-tasting fruit growing in Peru called camu-camu can contain as much as 3 000 milligrams of vitamin C for every hundred grams of its weight. Orange juice contains only 50 milligrams per hundred grams. Anyone convalescing from a protracted or severe illness needs approximately ten times more vitamin C than a comparatively healthy person. Do try to obtain this vitamin C from natural sources. It is absorbed by the body in the small intestine, so there is a limited time for it to be used and processed, and once this time has gone it rushes straight through and is excreted in the urine. This, to my mind, means that it is better to have your vitamin C spread in smaller amounts over shorter periods of time than to take a massive dose once a day. However, if you are really ill and your requirement for vitamin C trebles or quadruples you can take much larger doses and have them quite satisfactorily absorbed. Don't forget, one cup of rosehip tea or those few sprigs of parsley or that glass of fresh lemon juice can give you your vitamin C every day in a natural form.

VITAMIN D

A lot of young and middle-aged people think it their bounden duty in the summertime to change the colour of their skin from its natural pigmentation to a deeper brown. Each year as winter's blasts are replaced by summer breezes you will find row upon row of devout, determined sunbathers on beaches and river-banks catching what is referred to as a 'tan'. The one who achieves the deepest colour in the shortest time wins some sort of status value on the beach, and anyone who unwisely indulges to the point of appearing a bright lobster pink on Monday morning at the office is given the wooden spoon in the sun-tan contest. In countries like Australia that are blessed with a good solid quota of sunshine, it is quite possible, even in midwinter, to sneak up on your neighbours and friends with a little advanced tanning.

The tanning process does several things functionally and structurally to us. It increases the melanin pigmentation of our skins, and after tanning has reached the point where we can get no darker, a very sad thing happens to us functionally: we absorb no further ultraviolet rays through the skin and therefore manufacture no more vitamin D. It is a truism that once we have reached our deepest possible tan we no longer burn at all, a sign that we are no longer absorbing ultraviolet rays. Without sunlight on our bodies no natural form of vitamin D is available unless we introduce it in the form of oily fish, milk and egg yolks. But sunlight is one of the last blessings that is still free, and it makes more sense to get vitamin D in the natural way if you can.

We are much more aware now than our grandmothers were that sunlight is a good thing. The days when tiny babies were bundled up in umpteen layers of heavy clothing so that only their noses showed are gone: now our children are happily sunbathing from a few weeks old and absorbing vitamin-D-making ultraviolet rays to keep their bones growing sturdily. Back on those sunlit beaches we find all shades of tan ripening on all shapes and sizes of prone bodies as the ultraviolet pours freely down, making a substance called calciferol just undernearth the surface of the skin. Synthetic vitamin D is made by irradiating yeast with ultraviolet light, and in some countries cow's milk is also irradiated artificially to increase its vitamin D content. Those glass· bottles in which we buy milk, however, do not mean that our milk is absorbing more and more ultraviolet as it sits on our front step in the early morning. For glass and most of our building materials absorb ultraviolet light, and you cannot get vitamin D through a window or a glass bottle. It is a fat-soluble vitamin and is easily stored in the body, so it is not necessary to get some each day as it is with vitamin C and the B-complex group.

If you have vague aches and pain in your bones it may mean you are in the early stages of rheumatism, but it may also mean you have lacked vitamin D over a long period of time. Elderly folk whose bones are ageing along with the rest of their bodies have a greater need for vitamin D and should make sure they get out in the sunlight as often as possible. If you believe in covering your body so that only your hands and face show, if you have long periods of work in artificial light, or if you are a night worker, it is quite possible you are not getting enough free vitamin D; so you must pay for your way of living and have it as a food supplement. Small amounts of this vitamin are found in milk, egg yolks, and butter, and slightly larger amounts in some of the oily fish such as tuna, salmon, sardines, and herrings: we find that these sources of vitamin D figure largely on the menus of people living in cold northern and extreme southern parts of the world where the hours of daylight are short and the natural vitamin D is not so plentiful.

This vitamin is essential to stabilise the function of calcium and phosphorus in the body, so it follows that if we haven't enough of it we progress towards a disease common in our grandparents' day—rickets. During the Victorian era and earlier it was considered quite remarkable and peculiar to expose any part of one's body to the sunlight if it was possible to cover it up. Present-day trends have gone to the other extreme, and we expose as much as we possibly can as often as possible—with a variety of results ranging from deep, painful sunburn to skin cancer and, in some places, to in-carceration for indecent exposure! Somewhere in between these two extremes lies good health with adequate vitamin D.

It *is* possible to have too much of this vitamin, either naturally or synthetically. Since it regulates the calcium and phosphorus balance and metabolism, it is obvious that too much or too little of it is going to interfere with our use of those important primary elements. Excessive amounts of vitamin D can result in a malabsorption of the calcium and phosphorus in the body so that they are deposited in soft tissues—forming stones in kidneys and bladder and gall-bladder—or in arteries, resulting in hardening and calcifi-cation. I would hasten to say that this is not often the case, for our vitamin D intake is a pretty obvious one, and we would soon know if we had had too much of it naturally. But if we take it synthetically, as a supplement, this probability is to be reckoned with. The fish-liver oils of cod and halibut contain vitamin D, together with the vitamin A that is needed to enable the D to work most efficiently, and this natural source is the one most used as a dietary supplement. No one has yet produced conclusive data as to what quantity of vitamin D is the 'right' quantity for an adult or child or an elderly person, but it is not difficult to tell whether you are having too little or too much. If you do need a supplementary source of the vitamin, you will find that manufacturers (as required by law) show the standard average dose on the container, and this should be a guide. I am certainly not going to say either 100 000 units or 50 units is the right amount for you; but it has been found clinically that over 100 000 units of the *synthetic* vitamin can be damaging.

Vitamin D also regulates the condition of the teeth through its influence on the calcium metabolic function. If a pregnant woman has a natural supplement of vitamin D before her child is born it is much more likely that the child will have fewer problems with teething and a sturdier set of fangs to chomp through all the terrible food it will be faced with during its lifetime. There is another interesting correlation here: our teeth are getting weaker as our need to use them is getting less. How many foods do you eat that have to be chewed really hard and long these days? You would have to stop and think before making a list. Do you eat your carrots and celery raw? Do you work your way through a plateful of lightly cooked grain in a porridge in the early morning, or do you settle for bland foods that require little or no tooth work? It is no wonder that Nature is shrugging her shoulders and saying, 'Well, if you won't use the things, you can blooming well do without them.' Our teeth would not be so weak and give up the struggle so early if we worked them a little harder.

Like vitamin A, vitamin D is necessary for the health of our eyes. Our eye health appears to be regulated to some extent by the amount of light that enters our eyes and how we deal with that light. You know how difficult it is to look straight at the sun—a clear indication that this is not what we are supposed to do for our health. The amount of light our eyes can tolerate is nowhere near the amount the rest of our bodies can take: this is why so many of us must wear dark glasses when out in the sun for any length of time. I am neither for nor against the wearing of dark glasses, though I feel they have a cosmetic value in that we tend to frown and screw up our eyes when there is too much sunlight: this can cause muscular tension and tightness and therefore nerve stress, leading to headaches and eye strain. Be careful of sunbaking if you are very fair-skinned, with pale hair and pale blue eyes —your body is not able to absorb too much of the sun's rays at once.

If you lived here until you were 500 years old you might be able to do without your dark glasses altogether. Folk who live in tropical countries near the Equator with long hours of hot, fierce sunlight to contend with have skins that are naturally pigmented to a much darker shade than ours. Among the darkest of all skin pigmentations are those of the African and the Australian aboriginal, who live where blinding sunlight falls over vast dry areas, unrelieved by green vegetation, making it necessary and indeed natural for them to possess this comforting tolerance to sunlight. Can you imagine a fair-skinned, blue-eyed northerner living in and trying to acclimatise to such conditions without the aid of sunglasses, hats and protective clothing?

The Eskimos are an exception: they live close to the midnight sun, with a minimal amount of sunlight and daylight, and you'd imagine their bones would be ready to crumble away altogether from lack of vitamin D. But the reverse is the case—rickets is unknown in Eskimo communities because their diet is almost entirely based on oily fish, an excellent vitamin D source.

It is good that we no longer see so many of the deformities associated with a rachitic child—the squaring of the head shape, the enlarging of joints, and the bow legs and bent long bones, which remind us of Dickens and his half-starved, malnutritioned children groping about in the backblocks of London, in dark rooms and midwinter misery. It is a rare mother nowadays who does not know that her child in its early formative years of growth needs sunlight in common-sense amounts.

VITAMIN E

Sadly, it is no longer true that bread is the staff of life. There was a time when bread was just this, a staff, something to lean on to give you strength. That was in the good old days when bread was made at home or baked in the village ovens straight from the grain grown in the fields, and ground—perhaps the previous day or even that morning—into whole-meal flour ready for baking. Somewhere around the end of last century it was discovered by flour-millers that flour would not go stale or become rancid if part of the grain, the 'germ of the wheat', was removed early in the piece and the flour bleached to whiten and virtually 'kill' it. The wheatgerm is the part of the grain that affects the keeping qualities of flour, for it contains the seed of new life: unless it is returned to the earth to grow or is ingested in our daily food the wheatgerm decomposes so that other forms of life such as moulds and bacteria can thrive on it and keep up the life-cycle though in a different form.

Wheatgerm was always a bit of a trial to flour-millers, for it clogged up their machinery, being soft and rather flabby in texture. It was a great day for them when wheatgerm was processed right out of the picture in the name of efficiency and was sold for pig-food or mixed with bran and pollard and fed to the poultry. But it was a sad day for the humans at the other end of the transaction when the housewife bought bread from which the vitamin E and the vitamins of the B group had been neatly and completely removed. We are told that bread is now once again 'enriched' with added vitamins, but it is undeniable that it no longer has the nutritional value it formerly had as a staple article of our diet to be eaten every day. When the valuable life-carrying ingredient was removed from the bread we lost not only our vitamins B and E but some vitamin A and many minerals and trace minerals. Most medical men and nutritionists will now tell you to stay off bread or cut it right down, whereas in former times—and not so long ago at that—one or two slices of bread could be eaten at each meal with great nutritional benefit. The way to get back this priceless ingredient is of course to buy wheatgerm from the health store—fresh each week, if possible —to replace what is now no longer in bread.

Perhaps the prime function of vitamin E is its protective role in cell division. Whenever cells divide in the body—and it's happening all the time from conception to birth, in growth and in middle age and in old age as cells die and become fewer in number—vitamin E should be present to protect this division against any random defects. Many diseases spring from cells that have gone awry, and scientists investigating cancer and the body conditions that lead to cancer are now discovering what they call 'free radicals', which occur when cells divide in a manner that is not usual.

Vitamin E has another important function: it is often called the 'muscle vitamin' and it plays its part here by increasing the efficiency of the entire muscular system, especially that of the heart muscle. When sufficient vitamin E is found in the body tissues and bloodstream one does not need so much oxygen to perform one's tasks well. This has tremendous value in our overladen air and our stuffy cities, where we can't breathe the purer form of oxygen we can find in open country with natural vegetation all around us exuding its oxygen waste products.

You would think that anything that could improve our overall body health under the conditions we live in would be hailed as one of Nature's provisions to keep our race going.

Not so! You try asking your doctor whether he thinks you should have a vitamin E supplement and he will probably say, 'Well, it won't hurt you. If it makes you feel happy to take it, you might as well.' It is astonishing to find that doctors have to work out for themselves whether they believe vitamins in a supplementary form can help many types of disease conditions: they are taught so little in their training about *health*, and about what the bodies they are treating are running on every day in the form of fuel.

As an example of how people sometimes catch hold of a half-truth and insist it is the entire truth, authorities may tell you not to take iron with vitamin E and not to take oestrogen with it either. This *can* apply if both those substances are of the synthetic variety, for it is proven that synthetic iron can inhibit your vitamin E function just as the vitamin can inhibit the function of the iron; but it does not apply to their ingestion from natural sources. In that storehouse of Nature's goodies, parsley, we find broken every rule man has formulated as to what to eat with what. In this one fresh green package we find one of the most concentrated and powerful natural surces of vitamins and minerals. Parsley has an exceedingly high iron and vitamin E content. They do not fight with each other, and both assimilate completely. Natural oestrogen manufactured by the body is not only compatible with added vitamin E but the vitamin can indeed prolong the high levels of oestrogen past our present-day stopping points: it can have beneficial effects before or even during menopause, and can have the effect of delaying it somewhat because of the general good tone and good health of the entire system. Maybe you are only as old as you feel, but I would say that you are as old as the efficiency of your cell-division.

Vitamin E is protective not only of the body but of other vitamins. It would appear to be necessary for the complete use of other vitamins in foodstuffs or from natural food supplements, and it does its job by protecting them from oxidation so that they are completely assimilated in their pure state. It was only discovered and named as a vitamin in 1936, and a list of the diseased states it has been used to treat since then cover most of the serious illnesses, particularly of the degenerative type, mentioned in the textbooks. It has been used in treatments for circulatory diseases, for muscular wasting and atrophy, for diseases of the reproductive system, in skin grafts, and in treating bed sores and muscular wasting after long periods of immobilisation; it has been used for menstrual problems and prostate problems; and for diabetics vitamin E has proved to be necessary, because diabetics absorb and apparently need much more of it in their body tissues than normal people.

So from what foods can we best supply our bodies with adequate amounts of this magnificent vitamin that can ensure a youthful old age and a longer life with all faculties still going strong? Wheatgerm is still the best and the most available and cheapest source of vitamin E, but you can supplement this with sunflower seeds, pumpkin seeds, beans and peas; you can use soy oil or safflower oil or apricot-kernel oil on your salads, and you can get much of your vitamin E, if you are Scottish born and bred, in your oatmeal porridge every morning. Vitamin E is also found in liver, in butter, and in egg yolks—although these articles of food are not what they used to be. It would be interesting to compare the vitamin E levels from naturally grown vegetables and grains and from naturally raised animals with the vitamin E levels in their more artificially reared relatives.

Some researchers are asking whether vitamin E can be used protectively and even preventively against radiation damage. Since it does protect cells as they divide and multiply, and it has been used correctively to remove damage from old cells, its possible function in counteracting the effects of radiation could be well worth investigating—if only for the sake of our peace of mind as we read the newspaper headlines.

Much of the published literature on vitamin E deals with

its function in heart diseases and its role as the 'fertility' vitamin. It will only make you more virile, if you are a man, by taking some of the load off that overworked body of yours, and particularly off your heart and circulatory and muscular systems: you feel, and are, less exhausted, and so your sex life improves. If you are a woman and you are having difficulty in conceiving a child, or if you feel too tired to enjoy any sexual activity, then vitamin E can help. Giving its protective care to your cell regeneration, it dilates the blood vessels, and it contains anti-thrombin, which prevents blood-clots. And so your blood can make its way happily through healthy vessels, instead of moving sluggishly through tired arteries and veins. This is why vitamin E is taken by folk with varicose veins, with haemorrhoids, or with circulatory clogging such as we find with high blood pressure and high cholesterol levels.

If you are taking a supplement of vitamin E, it is essential to begin with no more than 100 milligrams per day for at least a week or two. If you suddenly dilate blood vessels and suddenly have fresh, clear blood coursing through them, you are going to put local strains on parts of the machinery. So you must be sure to increase your circulatory function slowly and steadily rather than give it a sudden boost that could be harmful and even fatal in extreme cases of weakness. Please don't get carried away and start yourself on enormous doses: ease yourself into taking it gradually and safely, and wait a few days or a few weeks for your general health to feel the effects.

Even old heart damage has been found to respond to some form of vitamin E treatment; but never attempt to treat yourself when such a vital part of your anatomy—the motor that keeps it running—is involved. Have yourself checked by qualified people who know what they are doing if you have any heart condition.

Do you have those brownish areas known as 'age spots' on your skin? Vitamin E has been used to help remove the wrongly programmed cells that cause them and to replace them with rightly wired cells that reproduce themselves correctly. If you have any condition that is slow to heal, such as varicose ulcers or skin eruptions; if you have severe tissue damage where cells are destroyed, as in a burn or an injury or a fracture, vitamin E taken internally can be used, together with a vitamin-E-based ointment externally—after your health adviser has found you free of infection and completed any localised treatment of the area.

This valuable vitamin is destroyed entirely when foods are fried and then frozen, so those TV dinners are not all they are cracked up to be. Any food that has been cooked, then frozen, then reheated is pretty low in vitamin E by the time it gets to your table, especially if fats or mineral oils are used anywhere in its processing. The best way to have a vitamin is to get it fresh from its primal source, in this case that germ of the wheat that holds the germ of life. If you wish to take a vitamin E oil and get your supplement this way, it is usually enough to have half a teaspoon or so straight from the bottle each day. Wheatgerm oil and sunflower oil and apricot-kernel oil are available in their cold-pressed forms, in which no heat has been applied to the grain at any stage of its processing.

Can you afford *not* to take vitamin E?

VITAMIN F

Do you know that your body manufactures cholesterol whether you have it in your diet or not? If you are told to go on a low-fat diet (which means a low-cholesterol diet) for a condition of obesity or heart disease or other associated disease states, you should know that as fast as you eliminate animal fats from your diet you ought to add vegetable fats (that is, vegetable oils), or you will be storing up more trouble than you had in the first place.

It may come as a surprise to you to be told that your body makes its own cholesterol. This is done in the liver, and if you have sufficient unsaturated fatty acids in your diet the cholesterol you manufacture can be handled very well and not stored against the walls of your arteries to cause you circulatory problems.

Now note this carefully: Any margarine or cooking oil that is solidified is usually hydrogenated, a process that destroys *all* the unsaturated fatty acid content. When you read on the label that there is such and such a percentage of unsaturated oil or fat in a margarine-type product, you should also be aware that it is very much better for it to be in a liquid or semi-liquid form than in a solid form. This is one of the anomalies that has arisen in the food industry as it has endeavoured to keep pace with the so-called nutrition experts who say that a diet high in animal fats leads to obesity and circulatory disease. But if only, *if only*, someone would proclaim that all those people without their animal fats, righteously losing weight at a great rate, should replace these fats with fats of *vegetable* origin so that the cholesterol manufactured each day in the liver will not just go on piling up against their arterial walls. Cholesterol cannot be processed and broken down and used in the bloodstream as it should be unless these unsaturated fatty acids are present in sufficient quantity to handle it. It's a matter of balance again: you can't remove one whole slab of dietary intake without compensating with another that will do the same job, and a far better one.

Vitamin F is often called lecithin, but it is not exactly correct to call it so because vitamin F as such appears to be a group containing the unsaturated fatty acids. Lecithin is certainly one of these, and its constituent, linoleic acid, is the part that handles your cholesterol balance. A deficiency of this vital component of our food can lead to a raised metabolic rate, and to overweight problems resulting from the non-processing of cholesterol; but even if you live on the most perfectly balanced diet otherwise, a lack of your vegetable oils can lead to underweight problems, too. This raised metabolic rate can also mean that your body is hurling all that food through itself at such a speed that you cannot absorb its components.

A deficiency of vitamin F, as well as leading to a raised metabolic rate, can lead to eczema, dull dry hair, and a nervous system whose impulses are very much awry. Kidney disorders can also occur, as well as impairment of the reproductive functions. It's a very vital group, this vitamin group that comprises the unsaturated fatty acids, and probably the most lacking in our diet unless we are conscious that we must have oils from vegetable sources (and from some animal sources like fish which have a slightly different method of assimilation in the body).

I believe that vitamin F is lacking to some extent in the diet of each one of us. Well, where can we get it from—which are the best sources? It exists as a group of fatty acids in soy beans with the oil from soy beans the highest source; in cold-pressed vegetable oils such as sunflower and corn and safflower and wheatgerm oil; it also exists in good quantities in oily fish such as eels, salmon, tuna, and the livers of codfish and halibut, and in turtles and two of the white animal meats, chicken and turkey. In my favourite rolled oats there is a large quantity of vitamin F: we'll meet this food again and again, more particularly in the chapter on food.

Vitamin F is also found in rice and in cornmeal and in wheatgerm itself, as well as in the oils from these grains. Those magnificent sweets prepared by Chinese and some Asian countries, candied watermelon seeds and rockmelon seeds, are exceedingly rich in vitamin F. Surely when we buy these fruits from our greengrocer we should stop and find a recipe somewhere that tells us how to candy the seeds to use as nibbles and appetisers before a meal, or as a talking-point finish.

The oils to be found in most nuts are high in vitamin F, so if you are a nut-eating vegetarian you are probably getting sufficient of this vitamin group. But bear in mind that cashew nuts are much lower in this vitamin than are most of the other common nuts we eat every day—or should eat every few days—such as almonds and brazil nuts. If you are a peanut fancier you will find vitamin F here too, although it is wise to keep your peanut intake not too high, since these nuts are slow to digest and very high in carbohydrate content and calorie value.

Vitamin F also plays a role in the correction of dandruff and acne, since it works within the fat-absorption system of the body. Your cold-pressed vegetable oils can be the way to regulate this over-activity in the sebaceous glands. It is thought that vitamin F also plays a part in regulating the thyroid gland.

The vitamin F group is destroyed by exposure to air over a long period and by the rancidity (or turning bad) of the vegetable oil or the animal fat in which it is found. This turning rancid, or oxidation process, happens through exposure to ultraviolet rays or to high heat. This is why it's so important that vegetable oil should be cold-pressed, and preferably sold in brown-coloured glass bottles to protect it from light. Nuts are better eaten raw, because the high temperatures of roasting or frying can destroy their vitamin F. When the oxygen present in the oils is heated it turns to peroxides, which are very toxic. It is therefore advisable to take vitamin E and vitamin F together so that the high intake of oxygen is sufficient to circulate around each human cell even if some deterioration has taken place in the oil or fat. It is next to impossible to have perfectly pure oils unless you tread out the olives with your bare feet and bottle the expressed oil immediately in brown glass and then store it in some deep, dark cellar away from all light; but you can mitigate the effects of light and heat by making sure that the oils you buy are clearly marked 'cold-pressed' and are marketed in brown or amber-coloured bottles, not in plastic.

This vitamin F group is vital to the continuing health of the cell membranes. If weakened from lack of this vitamin, they eventually rupture and the contents of the cells leak out and the cell dies. If enough of these chain reactions go on, the death of the cells that are not replaced can cause severe illness. If the cells are busy dying off in your heart muscle, your heart is not going to function as it should. Our youthfulness and resilience depend to a certain extent on the strength of the walls between each cell that provide the surface for vitamin C to work on, cementing each cell to another. Without vitamin C and vitamin F coming to us from our food or in natural supplementary form each day we are deliberately knocking down our cell walls with tiny sledgehammers of apathy and ignorance of our body's requirements.

In the case of my own body and its food preferences, I find I thoroughly enjoy an occasional meal of oily fish. When I set about preparing the evening meal, quite often my instincts say, 'Cold rice salad with salmon and chives and chopped green pepper, a little egg yolk boiled, and some parsley and kelp sprinkled over the top', or 'Tuna salad, with hunks of the sweetish brown flesh, and cottage cheese and pineapple wedges, mixed together and heaped on lettuce leaves with a few nasturtium leaves and perhaps dandelion leaves and a light dressing over the top of soy oil or garlic oil, with a little lemon juice and parsley sprigs.' My instincts are quite specific, aren't they? It's not often my stomach says 'turtle soup', but it most certainly says 'rolled oats' to me every single morning of my life.

If you are taking wheatgerm oil or pumpkin-seed oil for your vitamin E, you are getting at the same time your vitamin F, which is going to act with it and help it do its magnificent work of oxygenating cells and keeping muscles and circulation working exceedingly well. If you can simplify your sources of vitamins, you won't need to make it a task each day to get vitamins in your food or to get your natural vitamin supplements. One or two or three good food sources, such as yeast and wheatgerm and cod-liver oil, can give you pretty well your whole vitamin intake in a balanced, biologically compatible dose without too much bother and too much technicality.

VITAMIN K

Vitamin K is known as the blood-clotting vitamin and it is most important in haemophilia, and in haemorrhaging in childbirth. It plays a part in the prevention of strokes, and in the prophylactic treatment of people who have had strokes. Strokes are haemorrhages in blood vessels whose walls are weakened, so it's common sense to have vitamin K in some form if you have a history of haemorrhaging-type diseases.

This vitamin is made by the body in the intestinal tract to some degree, but it must be absorbed from the food as well. Green leafy vegetables contain lots of it, and so do wheat bran (the outside husk of the wheat) and wheatgerm (the seed of life within the wheat grain). If you have a disease of the liver, of the intestinal tract, or of the bile duct, this can cause a lack of vitamin K in the body. So you should make sure—for so many different reasons—that those green leafy vegetables are in a salad bowl on the table every day. Vitamin K is found in spinach and cabbage and carrot tops, and also in alfalfa, that wonderful alkaliser for those with high tissue-acid conditions such as arthritis. It is also found in soy-bean oil and cod-liver oil, those two potent carriers of vitamins that should be used more intelligently than they are to give us our daily vitamin quota.

Vitamin K is specially important for those of us who worry about chemical preservatives in our foodstuffs, though we may have little knowledge of their effects: for it can be used as a natural preservative to control fermentation in foods without bleaching them or causing them to lose any of their flavour. Researchers in America, planning how best to equip their spacemen with food, found that irradiation appeared to preserve it for long periods without any apparent damage. But later it was found that irradiation of food destroys all the vitamin K. So, unless our spacemen are to bleed to death when they bump themselves against the furniture, a better method of food preservation must be found. Surely vitamin K itself could be used to preserve the food so that there would be added amounts of it in the blood to combat the haemorrhage likely to occur under reduced outside pressure.

Vitamin K may seem relatively unimportant—for we all appear to get sufficient of it not to bleed to death each morning before breakfast. But when haemorrhaging does occur, as in prolonged and difficult childbirth or in blood complaints, the clotting factor it contains proves it to be a very important vitamin indeed.

VITAMIN P—Rutin

Rutin is only a part of vitamin P, but it seems to be the major part and the name is often used synonymously. You have probably heard of bioflavenoids in regard to vitamin C, and vitamin P appears to be the bioflavenoid part of this major vitamin. When you have a cold it is better to *eat* the lemon or the orange than just to drink the juice of the fruit, because the juice does not contain any of the bioflavenoid substances that are found in the white pith just underneath the skin. Rutin or vitamin P is valuable to sufferers from high blood pressure, for it strengthens and increases the efficiency of the small blood vessels—both the arterioles (the smallest of the arterial vessels) and the venules (the tiniest of the veins). If the blood pressure is high the 'pipes' the blood is going through must be as good and strong as possible to carry such a high pressure; and rutin can be used as a food supplement or in medicinal quantities to strengthen the wall of the small blood vessels.

Exposure of patients to X rays over prolonged periods can weaken the tiny veins and arteries in any part of the body.

Rutin can act as a preventative if you have enough of it in your diet. It's easy enough to come by if you eat berry fruits such as blackcurrants, cherries and strawberries, and lemons and grapes and grapefruit; and it is also found in plums— indeed in most fresh, raw fruit. And don't forget that it is better to eat a fruit than merely to drink its juice. The juice is certainly easier for the body to absorb, but you are throwing away all that vitamin P left in the drier cells of pith and skin of the fruit you have juiced.

Rutin is found in buckwheat, the commercial source of this vitamin, and it is also found in a herb plant called rue, from which it takes its name. Rue was the cheapest and most available source of rutin during the two world wars, when this vitamin was used to thin the viscosity of blood and promote diuresis, the expelling of fluid from body tissues. It was then found that the rutin also contributed to a drop in blood pressure, and it is now mainly used for this purpose. My patients who have high or fluctuating blood-pressure patterns are always treated with rue as one of their herbal mixture ingredients: the general affinity for the circulatory system that this plant has is quite astonishing in its immediate and lasting effects.

Rutin is also of great therapeutic value for diseases of the eye, even severe ones like glaucoma in which fluid build-up and engorgement of blood vessels are found.

The eyes are two windows of the body through which the condition of blood vessels can be observed. In my iridology work, studying patterns in the iris and in the sclera (the white of the eye), I can often diagnose circulatory disease conditions remarkably accurately from the open windows there before me.

Some remarkable improvements have occurred in patients with circulatory problems who have been given rutin as a supplement, but you can get this valuable and most necessary vitamin from those fruits I have mentioned, and from buckwheat which you can roast and add to your morning muesli:

you will have plenty of vitamin P to keep those blood vessels pumping away at their efficient best.

Never attempt to diagnose your own heart condition or that of any of your friends and family: this is a job for a qualified person—a medical man if you are medically minded or a practitioner whom you can trust if you are naturopathically minded.

What have we learnt from this discussion of vitamins? We should have learnt that we need only small quantities of them, but that without those small, sometimes infinitesimal, quantities available to us from our food or from food supplements we are going to be sick people indeed. They are vital—even their name implies that—and most of us know enough about them from popular literature to be conscious that if we have a cold we need more vitamin C and if our nerves are shot we may need more vitamin B complex.

We can simplify vitamins in one or two or three sentences. If you eat wheatgerm, yeast, fresh green vegetables and fresh fruits, and vegetable oils and some oils from fish, you should be getting sufficient vitamins to see you through. If you eat food that has been refined and processed and altered in its form and content, you are less likely to be getting your full vitamin needs supplied each day. If you hate salads and never eat raw fruit, and live on a diet of coffee, white bread and pies, then it means you could be well on the way to major disease from a total lack of vitamin material. You may hold out for years, feeling more miserable every day, but eventually vitamin deficiency will catch up with you to such an extent that you will have no vitality left to fight against disease. Now that you know, it's your own fault if you choose to be sick!

To feel vital and as alive as it is possible to feel when well nourished, you should make a mental list of a few simple foods that contain the vitamins you need for your physical maintenance and well-being. We need the minerals to lay the foundation, but the vitamins are the bricks and mortar that build us into living, walking, running, bounding-with-energy, healthy individuals. Once you have sorted out which food-stuffs bearing their load of vitamins you prefer to eat each day, then you can automatically include these food items and stop worrying about your vitamin balance. You must first *know* how to be healthy, then *do* what is necessary, and forget about it.

If you want to take your vitamins in tablet form, preferring to trust the manufacturer's label and his reputation, then this is entirely up to you. But I believe it is more aesthetically gratifying to sit down to a vitamin-rich meal with all its colourful fresh fruits and vegetables, with its nuts and fruit juices, with its grain products in wholemeal home-baked breads, than it is to pop twenty-odd pills into your mouth every morning at the breakfast table. Remember, the natural sources are always the best.

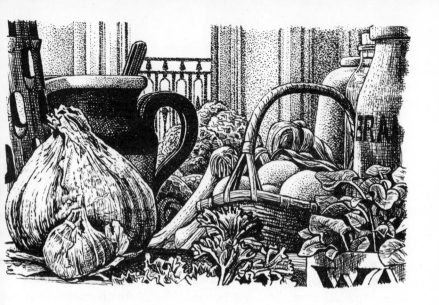

2

Mighty Minerals

I was once introduced to an experienced naturopath of many years' standing, a pioneer in the field of mineral treatments, as 'This is Mrs Hall, who has written a book on herbs.'

'H'mm,' was his assessment of this accomplishment. 'You know herbs only work because of their mineral content.'

He may be just about right, although I would quarrel with him as to whether that's the only reason herbal medicine works. Minerals control the body's chemical balance; homeostasis, it's techically called, an ideal state of physical equilibrium. In a fit body, sodium is balanced proportionately with potassium to keep kidneys functioning efficiently; calcium is balanced with sodium and phosphorus in the digestive processes; iron has with it the necessary tiny 'trigger' of copper so that oxygen can be available to the tissues via the bloodstream; a delicate mineral interplay ensures the efficiency of the automatic body processes, providing the framework in which vitamins, enzymes, and amino-acids, the chemical changers of foodstuffs into body fuels, can do their job. All the vitamins in the world can't help maintain or restore good health unless the mineral groundwork is present.

Let's look at cases. If a patient comes to me with finger-nails cracking, ridged and brittle, and says, 'I think I need calcium', my first response is, 'Why?' This does not endear me to the patient, who then has to do some thinking. Perhaps she has read it somewhere or the next-door neighbour has told her. It is possible to spend much money with the best possible intentions on a great variety of nutritional supple-ments and get no result whatsoever. Of course that woman needed calcium, but she needed silicon much more, so I prescribed for her tablets of *Equisetum arvense*, or horsetail, a strange little herb resembling asparagus, which has one of the highest natural silicon percentages to be found in all the plant kingdom—between 7.7 and 10 per cent—and which also contains calcium and sodium salts and iron in a biological-ly perfect balance for brittle fingernails. I trust my herb-mineral treatments, because nature has placed there in the plants the correct proportions compatible with animal and human metabolism. If that patient had taken only calcium it would certainly have helped her fingernails, but her body would have had to work harder than if she had the correct balance of the other minerals with the calcium to make it a perfect treatment.

If I diagnose a patient as needing iron and tell her so and she replies, 'Oh, I can't take iron, it makes me constipated', my next query is, 'Does parsley make you constipated?'

'Oh, well, no,' she'll reply, 'I've never noticed *that*.'

'Does watercress, does bran, does molasses, do avocados, make you constipated?'

'Oh, no, just the opposite.'

'Then you can take iron,' I tell her, 'for these foods contain iron with a difference, iron in correct biological balance with other minerals, vitamins and enzymes.'

This natural iron is in the form we can assimilate without side-effects; so a tired, anaemic, pale person with low vitality can eat parsley with its vitamin E, vitamins B and C, the digestive enzyme apiin, and its iron, potassium, copper, and magnesium, and assimilate the whole lot in one and a quarter hours—the fastest digestion time of any vegetable, fruit, nut or grain—without constipation resulting.

Watercress is another multi-vitamin and mineral combination to eat every day if possible. It has high percentages of calcium, sodium, magnesium, iron, phosphorus and chlorine, plus a goodly quota of vitamin A, B_1, B_2, niacin, and vitamin C. If you live in the country and have watercress growing naturally in creeks and streams, wash the stems thoroughly before eating—it can be a temporary lodging for the liverfluke parasite.

Talking of iron, brings me to copper, without which iron cannot be properly processed and utilised by the body. It needs only a minute 'trigger' of copper to fire off the iron assimilation process, but without it much of any iron present would pass through unused. This is often why faeces are dark or black when inorganic iron—that is, iron from synthetic sources—is prescribed. No evidence like this shows when organic or natural iron from natural vegetable sources is taken.

The foods containing this copper catalyst are many, but the best are leeks, garlic, parsley and broccoli, and, of course, watercress; and, of the more medicinal herbs, dandelion and red clover. Iron is the element that oxygenates or burns out body wastes and carries fresh oxygen to every body tissue, rebuilding and restoring its healthy function. So that little trace of copper is most important to start this constant re-birth cycle.

Phosphorus is important, too. The muscular, skeletal,

circulatory and nervous system all need phosphorus, and it combines with calcium in the metabolism of foods. It is a vital element in all body cells.

Dairy foods are high in phosphorus—one good reason for a balanced intake of cheese, butter, milk and eggs. But the adverse effects of our present-day pasteurised homogenised milk from cows fed with antibiotics and synthetic hormones, our cheese artificially 'matured' in half the time, our butter artificially coloured and salted, and eggs from hens fed synthetically under artificial daylight in battery cages, do much to make one wary of obtaining a phosphorus quota from dairy food sources.

These same dairy foods have a bad reputation for forming mucus in the body. Many books and articles have been written advising complete abstention from dairy foods. Certainly if you have a body that is loaded with mucus, with bronchial problems, with acid problems, with congestion and inflammation, you would not want to deal it another blow in the form of mucus-forming foods. But let me tell you that a healthy body will not form mucus no matter what food is eaten. Perhaps I had better qualify that last statement. If you live on bacon, eggs, six slices of white toast, marmalade and a glass of milk for breakfast every morning, this is tempting fate. Your body will most certainly complain and most certainly produce mucus. But if your diet is a balanced one with a little of everything, and your body is in a good state of health, then it will not produce mucus but will eliminate the waste products through skin, lungs, kidneys and bowel.

Minerals are the structural framework of the body, the foundations of its ability to live. And all the vitamins in the world, all the enzymes and amino-acids, could not give us the necessary food supplements to replace the basic minerals that provide the structure on which they work.

Minerals are usually heavy elements, and when our land is cultivated or desecrated to the extent it now is in all parts of the globe the topsoil, where most of our life comes from, is often either completely removed or buried under layers of macadam, concrete, and buildings. The minerals that used to be available to us indirectly in our everyday diet through plants and crops naturally grown are no longer there in the topsoil. Such natural heavy minerals as iron—particularly in its phosphate form, which is how it is mainly needed by the body—have been washed out of topsoils and mined out of subsoils and leached by chemical action. Sadly, much of our valuable natural iron is at the bottom of the continental shelf, under the ocean. It is no longer replaced by the death and decay of plants and animals, by the natural chemical change and regrowth taking place in the topsoil; and we have to add it artificially to many of our pastures to get them to grow anything at all.

When Nature is left alone the correct balance of minerals is available to every form of life through its habitat and its foodstuffs. But a natural environment is not easy to find any more. Now we have to think about the mineral earthworks of our bodies, to find out whether we are lacking in one or another of these vital elements, and to take steps to see that we get them, either through dietary control or by using natural mineral supplements.

There are many signs by which the trained naturopath or biologist or biochemist can tell whether any particular minerals or mineral groups are lacking in the diet; and it is best to seek expert advice. Though many magazines and newspapers give information that enables the layman to learn something about his body, this is only general information. Each person is entirely different, and requires variations within a standard general treatment for any condition. You may be quite happy eating your daily ration of kelp or going on a famous nutritionist's diet of vitamin B_6 and lecithin, or you may live to a ripe old age convinced that cabbage and potato water contain enough minerals for your daily ration. But it stands to reason that if you are a child of ten playing football, or a pregnant woman with three other children, or an elderly retired bank manager suffering from rheumatoid arthritis, there will be tremendous variation in the dosages of the minerals required. Natural mineral supplements will not be detrimental to your health if they are taken in the quantities and the manner prescribed on their labels, for much research and experience has gone into their preparation. But each of us is sufficiently different from everyone else (thank God!) for his body to have its own special needs that can be diagnosed by a trained nutritionist.

Apart from this, the mineral requirements of your body differ from time to time and from circumstance to circumstance. If you are trying to fight off a cold (we shall deal with colds later) you are going to need heavy, prolonged dosages of iron and calcium and magnesium for several days in a particular combination that will aid your body's 'fight-back' mechanism to work more efficiently. If you are a nursing mother, your need for calcium of course is great; and if you are pregnant that need is even greater. The unborn child is taking from the mother's body as much calcium as it needs and leaving her with only the remainder, so that if her calcium intake is not sufficiently boosted she will suffer such ailments as dental decay, bone degeneration, and under-activity of the digestive apparatus.

CALCIUM

The human body has more calcium in it than any other mineral, and about 90 per cent of this calcium is in the bony structure and the teeth. This calcium has to be progressively renewed, and it takes about six years for it to be renewed completely. If sufficient of the mineral is not absorbed during this time degenerative processes take place at a much faster rate, particularly in the skeleton, from which reserve store calcium is first withdrawn if a serious lack of it persists. The remainder of the calcium, the 10 per cent or so, is used in the metabolic processes of the body, in particular those of digestion; and it is also used by the parathyroid glands in a balancing or controlling action that affects the metabolic rate.

It is obvious, then, that if you are not taking sufficient calcium in your everyday diet your digestion will suffer. This is why many medical practitioners advise their stomach-ulcer patients to drink large quantities of milk. Milk is certainly a source of calcium, but it's rather difficult for the stomach to process and digest, and it is useful mainly because its fatty content may line and cover the ulcerated area of the stomach, thus fooling it into thinking it is better than it is. Calcium is certainly used in the treatment of ulcerated areas in the intestines, but it must be given in a form that is easily and readily absorbed.

A recent American survey revealed that 85 per cent of the population groups tested were deficient in calcium to either a minor or a major degree. Calcium cannot function alone without other supportive substances such as phosphorus and magnesium and vitamin D, which stimulate the calcium absorption; but it would be beyond the scope of this book to attempt to explain all these overlapping patterns. We'll just deal with calcium on its own—as long as you bear in mind that nothing in nature ever stands on its own.

Here are some of the functions of your everyday living in which calcium plays a tremendous basic role: It is necessary during pregnancy and lactation, and it is equally necessary in the early years of a child's life when bone and teeth formation takes place at its greatest rate. Calcium is also necessary for elderly people, and lack of it can disrupt the enjoyment of their later years. Calcium is needed for the proper processing of all the vitamins in our foodstuffs; and, by way of a return for services rendered, vitamin D then stimulates calcium's own absorption. Calcium plays a big role in the health of the heart muscle and the nerves associated with it; and, having an alkaline reaction in the body, it controls the acid-alkaline balance. It stimulates the activity of enzymes, and indirectly, because of all these other activities, it increases the general resistance of the body to disease.

Lack of the right kind of readily absorbable calcium in the diet can lead to dental decay, rickets, and other associated bone diseases, to degeneration of the function of the heart as a major muscle of the body, and to a general impairing of the metabolism to the point where perhaps you don't feel really ill but you can't recall ever feeling really well.

Many patients I see with an obvious calcium lack—confirmed by their dietary habits and by physical and biological signs—are living on reserves they do not have. They are trying to force an engine that is failing in power up grades that are too steep for it to handle. Often these patients are chronically tired, and no wonder either, because they are running like mad to stay on the one spot. When sufficient calcium is returned to a body that is craving for it, there is a gradual improvement in condition and tone until that person, for the first time in perhaps many years, feels what it is like to be healthy.

The highest calcium content of any food is to be found in parmesan cheese. So why don't we all just have a supplement of parmesan cheese every day and leave it at that? Because we must also consider how easy it is for the body to absorb. Next on the list in calcium content come sesame seeds, and here we're onto a winner among good foods. Sesame seeds have a unique mineral balance amongst the grain or seed foods in that they contain twice as much calcium as phosphorus; most grains are high in phosphorus and low in calcium, so sesame is valuable with its correct biological balance of these minerals in roughly the same proportions as they are needed in the body. It follows that sesame seeds are easy to digest. I am not going to tell you how much sesame seed you should eat every day, or every week for that matter, for this will vary with your own dietary and culinary habits. And you may or may not like the taste. But I shall tell you that in every hundred grams of sesame there are approximately

1 025 milligrams of available calcium. (Egg yolks have somewhere between 120 and 250 milligrams of available calcium in every hundred grams of their weight.) Swiss cheese, renowned the world over as one of the purest and most highly concentrated sources of animal calcium, has about 1 020 milligrams of calcium per hundred grams of its weight. The foods mentioned on following pages will give you an idea of which ones you can include each day to maintain your calcium reserves.

Cabbage, particularly the outside green leaves, gives you more calcium than cream cheese and about three times more calcium than cow's milk. Have coleslaw as often as you can. especially during the hot weather when you don't really feel like large amounts of cooked food: just rip off those outside leaves of the cabbage, and chop and slice until they are reduced to fine shreds that will not overload your stomach. Add some shredded carrot and grated onion and a few chopped chives and some of your favourite soya mayonnaise. Many people say, 'Oh, all that raw stuff gives me wind!' 'Of course,' I reply. 'It's because you don't have enough calcium.' They don't think I'm serious; but it's a fact that if you have enough calcium available to your digestive system you should not have any flatulence after eating raw foods.

Raw cabbage should be able to be taken by anyone in small quantities with no discomfort whatever, but until the stomach linings are in a healthy, resilient and chemically balanced state, discomfort may result. If this is so, you may put your cabbage through the juicer, not forgetting to include those precious darker green outside leaves with their high proportion of minerals and vitamins. But always bear in mind that cabbage juice should be drunk immediately after it is freshly pressed. Any juice from any vegetable or fruit loses much of its organic nature when it is stored: oxidation takes place with every passing minute, and deterioration ensues rapidly. Cabbage juice has been used extensively in the treatment of gastric and duodenal ulcers because of its high calcium content and its vitamin C, both healing agents for the intestinal mucosa.

Calcium, in higher or lower quantities, is found in all green leafy vegetables, such as broccoli, spinach, endives, lettuce, and brussels sprouts.

Kelp contains abundant free and easily assimilable calcium, and so does Irish moss. These seafood or rather sea-flavoured vegetables can be included as often as you enjoy them, or they can be taken in therapeutic quantities if your calcium levels are truly low. Soya beans, those gifts to every vegetarian, rank high on the list also, and calcium is only one of their many attributes. Parsley, as well as its vitamin content, is beautifully rich in minerals, and calcium is one of them. Dandelion greens, watercress, and horseradish are three more of the herbal contributors to your optimum calcium levels. If you believe as I do that honey is one of the gifts of the gods to us, then you will be pleased to know that honey helps to retain calcium in the body.

Molasses is another good source of calcium, which I'll deal with more fully when we speak about iron. Almonds, which are amongst the alkaline foods, are also calcium carriers: they have a beautiful balance of calcium, phosphorus and magnesium plus other useful ingredients. Their protein value is high, and they contain more of their mineral quota if you eat them with the skins on.

Buttermilk and yoghurt are preferred sources of calcium in the dairy-food group. Any milk that has been cultured with bacterial growth has also been partially digested, so the fatty content is changed and the protein more readily assimilated than in uncultured milk and dairy products. Yoghurt deserves a whole chapter to itself, and we shall speak of it when we talk about good food sources; but I mention it here for its calcium value and, in particular, its ease of digestibility.

Natural bran is another food on our list. This outer husk of the wheat has not only a good calcium component but contains phosphorus and magnesium and even silicon, and it not only has a healing action on the bowel and abdominal walls but improves the muscular tone, increasing peristaltic action and relieving the constipation that can accompany many diseases.

It is interesting that Asian and Oriental people seldom exhibit calcium deficiency symptoms, though their diet does not always contain good sources of this mineral. Genetic tests have shown that people of Oriental and Asian descent need less calcium in their bodies than do those of fair skin and European extraction. Why this is so has not been clearly indicated by any of the researchers whose published work I have read. The general opinion is that human beings are amongst the most adaptable creatures, and that Asian diets low in calcium have produced a race that does not need it chemically as we do. Smaller and slighter in their bony skeleton, Asians can remain apparently healthy on diets we would regard as nearly at malnutrition level. Some studies suggest that later generations of white Caucasians may be born with less need for calcium than we have as they acclimatise themselves genetically in advance to foodstuffs that may not have even the partially denuded quality of those we enjoy here and now. The feeding of the world's inhabitants is going to be a major task, and my optimistic belief is that Nature is not only working with us but ahead of us—or even in spite of us—to alter our requirements in accordance with what will be available to us.

PHOSPHORUS

Phosphorus is often found in conjunction with calcium in related body processes, and both elements occur very often in the same foods. Phosphorus affects the nervous and mental state of the human organism, though 90 per cent of it is found in the bones. The phosphorus in the body is renewed much faster than the calcium, replacing itself completely about every three years. Phosphorus is an acid-forming mineral, and its happy combination with calcium tends to produce a neutral environment and a state of equilibrium. They balance each other, and proportional amounts of both are needed before either can react at all. Vitamins of the D, C and A groupings are also necessary for the full and complete use of the phosphorus compounds in the body. Most of these are called lecithins and are found in many different parts of the body: in tissues and lymph glands, in many body fluids, and in the white matter of the nerves and the grey matter of the brain (the main centres of their function). The reason why some form of phosphorus is included in so many diets and tonic mixtures and food supplements is that all our body's functions are controlled initially by our nervous impulses.

The phosphorus and calcium partnership is a mutually dependent system in which one supplies what the other lacks, one is weak when the other is strong, one is giving when the other is receiving. It is like the natural balance of *yin* and *yang*, of positive and negative, of male and female, that is essential for life to begin and to continue—and to achieve harmony.

I often find amongst my patients young women with an acid condition of the vagina (an infection or inflammation or irritation) that is most happily and naturally corrected by the male sperm. Female vaginal secretions are generally acid, and the male secretion has just the correct alkaline balance to produce a neutral state for both. So intercourse has a neutralising, stabilising, balancing effect on both male and female in every possible way—chemical, emotional and spiritual.

So our ration of calcium and its related and (to a certain extent) opposite ration of phosphorus are working inside us to achieve metabolic equilibrium. Calcium is at the receiving end, while phosphorus gives the stimulus through its positive action on the nerve impulses and many of the mental functions that distinguish man from plant and animal. Phosphorus is necessary for the processing of carbohydrates and fats, and it combines with calcium to do this essential job. It is found in all body cells, and it stimulates enzyme action for the turning of fuel into substances the body needs in regulated amounts to function at all. It has a tonic effect on the circulation; and when this is poor, as in low blood pressure or sluggish functioning of the heart muscle, it can play a very important part therapeutically.

Phosphorus conditions the nervous system so that its responses are clearer and less affected by the stresses that wear away the nerve insulation and give us bare telephone wires instead of healthy, properly responding communication tracks. The condition of skin and hair and fingernails is also governed by phosphorus; and although other elements such as calcium and silicon are basically needed, phosphorus must be there also to keep the nerve supply to these areas at its peak performance.

Phosphorus deficiency shows up in many subtler ways amongst which are loss of weight and general debility, and limited growth and defective bone and teeth formation in children. And phosphorus is often sadly lacking in the bodies of people who 'live on their nerves'. You all know them— those stressful, highly strung, tense, usually over-active people who burn off every ounce of fat and stay thin and trim to the envy of their plumper friends. They need more phosphorus than others because their nerves are over-functioning and constantly in use, and they can very easily become victims of phosphorus starvation. We need these people to get things done in the world: they fly about and organise and do and achieve; others rely on them when projects need to be undertaken and problems solved. But their nerves (and therefore their whole physical structure) suffer severely with the stresses put upon them. Such people are usually oversensitive and feel very deeply the obligations and the challenges they face; and the nervous system takes the brunt of the attack. They can be helped by eating foods rich in phosphorus to counteract to some extent their body's excessive demand for it.

Foods that are rich in vitamins are usually found to be

fairly low in mineral content, and phosphorus is one of the first of the minerals to disappear from the scene when the vitamin content is high. The greatest general source of phosphorus is to be found in seeds and grain foods. All the wholegrains and the beans and nuts are very rich in it, and these foods should be required dietary items every day so that sufficient phosphorus is always available. As with all natural fuel substances, any excess will be thrown off naturally and not stored to create harmful waste. Phosphorus is also found in dairy foods; but these foods are not what they used to be and it is wise to get the bulk of your phosphorus from vegetable sources.

Wheatgerm is one of the richest sources of phosphorus, containing approximately one gram in every hundred grams of this food. That's a mighty high percentage of mineral; so, as a guaranteed early-morning source of phosphorus, we should have wheatgerm sprinkled on our breakfast cereal or on our fruit breakfast. The bran, the outer husk of the wheat, is also a good source of phosphorus.

Brazil nuts and almonds are amongst the highest in phosphorus content of the nut range of foods, and their pleasant taste and high protein value make them first choices for something to nibble on. Oatmeal, with its balanced calcium and phosphorus levels, is another grain high on the list. The lentil soup that was one of my grandmother's specialities contained lots of phosphorus, for she threw in not only lentils but barley and onions and some whole wheat, and just before serving she sprinkled parmesan cheese over each plate. Parmesan contains about one gram of free phosphorus per hundred grams of the cheese.

Pumpkin seeds are excellent sources of this mineral and, like wheatgerm, they are exceptions to the rule about vitamin and mineral content not being found at high levels in the same food. They can be bought from your health store in several different varieties: the Mexican pepitas, which are the seeds from a particular South American variety of pumpkin, or the plain old yellow pumpkin seeds that we scrape out and throw away (into the compost heap, I hope) before we steam pumpkin as a vegetable. If you'd rather give yourselves the benefit instead of the compost heap, wash the seeds carefully and spread them out to dry on sheets of paper, on a hot, sunny day when the humidity is low. The seeds can then be stored in a glass jar and used as nibbles or quick snacks. Or do as I sometimes do—I have a jar of assorted herb seeds, vegetable seeds and dried fruits in my car so that if I have no time for a meal I can chew little handfuls of seeds and nuts and fruits.

Sunflower seeds have similar properties. These are the elongated, greenish kernels from the seeds of the common sunflower plant, that enormous yellow dish of sunshine that we hardly ever see growing now. Plantations of this flower are cultivated in the Baltic countries and in Russia, and wherever farmers are realising its value commercially. The seeds can be processed and the sunflower oil extracted from them to use in cooking and in salad dressings and as a medicinal oil to be taken internally for its vitamin E and phosphorus content. Sunflower seeds can also be sprinkled over muesli or stewed fruits, or on dried fruits that have been soaked overnight in a little water; or they can be eaten just as you buy them from your health store. The soft green kernels have a characteristic flavour that blends well with other seeds and dried fruits.

Sesame seeds have a balance of calcium and phosphorus that is not typical of seeds and that gives them special value. They should be kept in a big glass jar in your kitchen, handy to be thrown on top of or into every possible dish, savoury or sweet, or on top of bread, biscuits and buns, into casseroles and vegetable hot-pots, into sweets made from dried fruits and stewed fruits, and they can even top a fresh fruit salad (sprinkled over a dash or two of yoghurt). Use sesame seeds in every possible combination with every possible food.

The soya bean is a phosphorus source that has been tapped

medicinally and is now becoming popular and prescribed in various diets as lecithin. There are many and various types of lecithins (phosphorus compounds), but the lecithin from soya beans is easily extracted, readily available, and comparatively cheaper than that from other sources. You should add soya beans to your diet if your nervous system needs a large intake of phosphorus.

Beans and lentils can give variety to the general diet, and are useful sources of phosphorus. Mung beans, so well known in Chinese cookery as sprouted bean shoots, are rich in phosphorus, as indeed are all sprouted seeds, and richer in their sprouted condition than they are when dry. Brown rice gives you plenty of phosphorus, and so do millet and rye. Kelp in all its shapes and forms is a good source, too.

The first of the herbs to appear on the phosphorus list is a favourite of mine—garlic. Garlic makes its presence felt internally and externally, and however you may feel about it you certainly can't ignore it.

Lychees, so beloved of the Chinese, and served so often to end a savoury meal as a delicate, sweet finale, are a good phosphorus food, and so are the water chestnuts that you may have eaten sliced and sizzled earlier in the meal. Chinese cooks, whether educated to our Western ways of thinking or not, still rely on food combinations that have been found nutritious for many thousands of years. They are adept at balancing one food with another to get the maximum dietary value from the combinations of elements found therein.

Mushrooms contain phosphorus and so do sweet corn and artichoke hearts. The sweet potato, not as widely used as it should be, is also blessed with phosphorus in appreciable amounts; and the ordinary potato (cooked in its skin, of course) contributes its humble share. In an interesting group in the dried fruits section peaches head the list, followed by apricots, bananas, raisins, prunes, dates and pears. Dried fruits, for the minerals and vitamins they contain, are amongst the best of our foodstuffs.

The green leafy vegetables come much lower down the list in phosphorus content, and so do fresh fruits, such as apples, pears, crabapples, lemons, grapefruit, oranges, and pineapple (the lowest of all). Vegetarians and people who adhere as closely as they can to a fruit-only diet should be aware that their phosphorus levels are in danger of being too low to enable their nervous systems to cope with everyday stresses. If you want to sit under the bough and eat bunches of cherries and grapes, that's OK; but don't try to work a forty-hour week and live only on fruit and fruit juices. A fruit diet is very well suited to slower life-styles, particularly in tropical climates where fruit is in abundance; but in more temperate conditions and with busier living patterns fruit and fruit alone will not do.

Phosphorus deficiency means lack of resistance to infections and can contribute to loss of mental and physical efficiency. Phosphorus is therefore necessary not only for athletes who must be in prime condition but for all of us, as preventive medicine, so that our natural immunity or 'fight-back' mechanism will be always ready to repel bacterial or viral invasion. Everything from noises in the head to shyness can receive benefit from an increased intake of phosphorus and its compounds. Phosphates of calcium and magnesium and sodium seem to be compounds readily assimilated, and naturopaths prescribe them to combat phosphate deficiency.

We have dealt with phosphorus on its own; but, like calcium and the other elements, it interacts and counter-balances, adjusts and co-ordinates with other minerals before it is assimilated by the body.

SODIUM

Sodium and potassium work in harness, just as calcium and phosphorus do. The sodium/potassium ratio is best seen in the functioning of the kidneys, that vital pair of filters that see to the removing and exchanging of chemical waste matter from tissues, from lymph and circulation, and to its excretion from the body. If your sodium/potassium balance is not correct your kidneys will be unhappy. Sodium and potassium together control most of the fluid interactions in the body, sifting, through cell membranes, foodstuffs and waste products. The sodium reaction chemically in body fluids is alkaline, and it is needed in every cell so that the osmotic pressure in body fluids and in the cells themselves is stabilised.

A good example of osmotic pressure is when you put salt on a snail or slug, and you watch the poor creature's body fluids exuding in a bubbly, frothy mess, leaving it dehydrated and very, very dead. Similar dehydration or, conversely, retention of body fluids, can occur if the sodium/potassium osmotic pressure balance is tipped either way.

If you haven't enough sodium you will not retain sufficient of your body fluids and will urinate excessively and, in extreme cases, become dehydrated to a dangerous level. If you have too much sodium the opposite may happen; you may retain body fluid in the tissues and put on more and more weight until your ankles swell and your tissues become flabby, your stomach protrudes, and your eyes almost pop out. Severe cases of fluid retention are just as dangerous and debilitating as their opposite condition of dehydration—the drying-out of body tissues and organs—that causes constipation and congestive headaches and every other sign of dryness. This sodium/potassium balance must therefore be correctly tuned.

One of the chief miscreants in the fight against overweight illnesses is common salt, sodium chloride. Every gram of salt holds to itself 70 grams of water in the body. Excessive salt in cells and tissues attracts and retains fluid, increasing your weight and size and making you feel flabby and congested and tired and miserable. Yet sodium is a very important element because it is necessary to alkalise and sweeten the digestive tract, and lack of it in a natural form can result in the over-acid conditions in which arthritis occurs.

I firmly believe that arthritics are born and not made. I have never yet had an arthritic patient who was not a person who suppressed his angers and frustrations and stresses, went bravely on doing his duty, and never let the side down. If you look at health as a whole picture of a whole person, you will see how this burying of 'acid' emotional reactions can trigger off or complicate an acid condition of the body tissues. Sodium in its compounds, particularly the sodium phosphate and sodium sulphate found in many natural sources of this element, can combat and neutralise such acid states if someone recognises this type of person in time. A naturopath who uses iris diagnosis (iridology) will know very well the picture an acid eye gives of the person being examined. Such a person battles on, saying, 'Don't worry, you go out and enjoy yourselves, I'll stay and do the dishes'; he fights to preserve the picture of a nonchalant, happy-go-lucky, able soul, coping well with his problems. But once you see that whitish-blue or greenish-blue acid eye confronting you under your magnifying lens, you know that the patient is not coping with his problems—he is burying them.

The natural release of stress and strain—whether by throwing dinner-plates, or abusing the missus, or getting drunk and disorderly—will ensure that you don't become arthritic! We all need some self-control; but if you can release your stress in some acceptable fashion you will not corrode in your own acid. I shall discuss arthritis later on. Its increasing frequency is a sign that our society does not provide sufficient outlets for the release of everyday tension, or else that our conditioning and training have inhibited these release processes. Medical authorities warn that smoking is a health hazard: they should also warn that salt is a weight hazard and can precipitate an arthritic pattern that will remain with the patient for the rest of his life. In so-called primitive societies where salt is not used but sodium is acquired from its vegetable sources, there is a low incidence of every complaint from cancer downwards. Heart disease appears to be less, high blood pressure is relatively unknown, and obesity is unheard of. Mind you, overweight problems can come from many other sources—such as under-activity of the thyroid gland, hormonal imbalance conditions, and even heredity; but when the salt intake is lowered some appreciable benefit can always be observed.

If you haven't enough natural sodium in your diet you may have digestive problems, particularly those associated with the incorrect or under-active functioning of your liver. The average daily need of sodium is about 8 to 10 grams, but the right amount for different people varies tremendously. Sodium is abundant in many green leafy vegetables and other foods, and your body will take natural sodium without retaining excess in fluids. Sodium plays a role in keeping the blood-plasma level at its required proportion, thus preventing the blood from becoming too thick through lack of fluid content. It is indispensable if we are to remove carbon dioxide efficiently, and it also is essential in keeping the calcium and magnesium salts in the fluid condition necessary for their absorption. When free calcium and magnesium are not correctly balanced and controlled in a fluid state, an arthritic condition can insidiously build up and be difficult to reverse once the calcium has been deposited in joints and bones. Foods high in sodium are top priority for anyone with arthritic or rheumatic symptoms, the alkaline reaction of the sodium salts buffering the high acid level in tissues and body fluids.

Sodium has been called the youth element. Sufficient free natural sodium in the diet can preserve suppleness and ease of movement, and help to keep the degenerative processes of old age at bay. The Hunza people whose normal life-span is over a hundred years, live in close proximity to streams and creeks where the natural sodium content is exceedingly high. The old folk in this community group are given another food rich in the youth elements of sodium and associated calcium and potassium—whey. While the old folk drink the whey, the children are given the curds—the solid part of the separated milk—where most of the natural calcium is found. The simple dietary knowledge, or the instinctive choice of natural-living groups such as this one shows us how well instinct can still function for our survival. If you wish to retain your youth and the suppleness of joints and muscles and ligaments, make sure your diet contains a goodly assortment of sodium-rich foods.

Kelp heads the list. It is not surprising that most of the salt substitutes to be found on shelves at your health store are composed mainly of kelp. There are up to 3 grams of sodium in every hundred grams of kelp, an exceedingly high concentration of this mineral in a readily absorbable form. You only need to look at the lithe, supple bodies of Japanese athletes and Thai dancing girls, and the magnificent posture and carriage of Malaysians and Indonesians, to see what a high sodium diet can do to preserve flexibility and prevent stagnation and degeneration of muscular tissue and joint movement. All these ethnic groups include seaweed in their general diet, particularly the Japanese, who have dozens of different types, shapes, colours and forms of seaweed products to choose from, mostly in a dried state. I like to sprinkle granulated kelp over my food on all possible occasions. It blends very well with rice dishes and with vegetable flavours (being a sea vegetable itself). This type of addition to the meal builds up sodium levels the easy way. Beat that sodium deficiency before it beats you: get in first and *prevent* creaky joints and aches and pains and acidity and such associated miseries. If you left out all the other minerals in kelp and used it only for its sodium content, it would still be close to the top of the list as one of Nature's good-est of good foods.

Olives come next best in sodium content, particularly the green variety. Nibbling a few ripe olives before your meal not only activates your taste buds and sharpens your appetite but increases the flow of saliva, and of bile and juices from the pancreas. This is another fringe benefit provided by natural sodium: it stimulates these digestive juices, increasing their enzyme content and activity, and thus taking some of the load off your stomach because the food is well prepared for digestion by the time it gets there. I don't know if you have ever eaten New Zealand spinach, the succulent and prodigal plant that grows like a weed and is often mistaken for one, and falls into the top category amongst vegetables for its high sodium content. I like to eat it fresh, picked straight from the plant just before it goes into the salad bowl; but it can be lightly steamed if you prefer it this way. The leaves have the unique spinach flavour, but in a milder form; and the plant, nothing like ordinary spinach in appearance, trails its juicy stems and soft, pale-green leaves all over any nearby support. Get some if you can, and include it often in your green salad bowl.

Now we come to what is really the food closest to my own heart—celery. Whenever I feel jaded about what to eat for lunch, or sick of the sight of fruit salad and peppermint tea and wholemeal bread, my thoughts turn always to celery, for me the most refreshing and completely satisfying food of them all. In experiments conducted by American dietary analysis groups, food values are recorded numerically as 'life energy units'. Celery is beaten for top place only by watercress and sugarbeet greens. It is a fast-growing vegetable with a high water content, and it has almost the exact balance of sodium and potassium needed to keep any pair of kidneys functioning at their most efficient level. My usual approanh to a meal of celery is to cut several stems, chop them up into handleable lengths, and fill the hollows with cottage cheese and a variety of toppings—yoghurt powder, walnut pieces, powdered dandelion leaves (which I have from a secret source of supply and have never yet seen on the market), a chopped date or two, or any other tasty morsel I can pick from amongst my edible herbs or find in my kitchen cupboard. Celery is always included amongst the foods I prescribe for arthritic patients, and I often find that they not only like it but have had a craving for it since their arthritis began. Just another instinctive eating pattern: your body knows what's best for it and sends you a loud, clear signal.

Horseradish can be classed as either a herb or a food, and it has the virtue of increasing the efficiency of the kidneys. It can be a boon to people who suffer from excess mucus in the system, for it not only contains the sodium/potassium combination but has a strange affinity for mucous linings throughout the body. This is why horseradish is prescribed for sufferers from sinusitis and hay fever. The horseradish stimulates and tones the soft mucous linings in sinus and antrum passages so that over-production of mucus may no longer occur, and the efficiently functioning kidneys both balance and then excrete the waste products.

And now that green friend of many blessings again, this time under its sodium heading—dandelion greens. What an absolutely complete food this little weed provides, with its sodium, its potassium, and its vitamins!

Watercress is not only highest on that life-energy scale we just spoke of, but turns up here too for its sodium content. If you know of creeks and streams where watercress is growing, pick it and use it at every possible opportunity. It can be difficult to grow under home garden conditions, demanding a constant supply of running water over its roots.

Parsley is like celery and watercress—it keeps on turning up, now for its sodium, though it could be found listed under almost any other mineral you care to name. Carrots, too, contain sodium, and, for me, share top billing with celery for the amount of minerals and vitamins they contain.

Most of the dried fruits such as figs, raisins, apricots and peaches are high in sodium content, and one of the most economical and versatile sodium sources—brown rice—can be combined with dried fruits to produce a variety of exotic sweet dishes. Brown, or unpolished, rice is one of the easiest of foods to prepare and can be mixed with sweet or savoury accompaniments in unlimited ways. Fresh coconut meat—

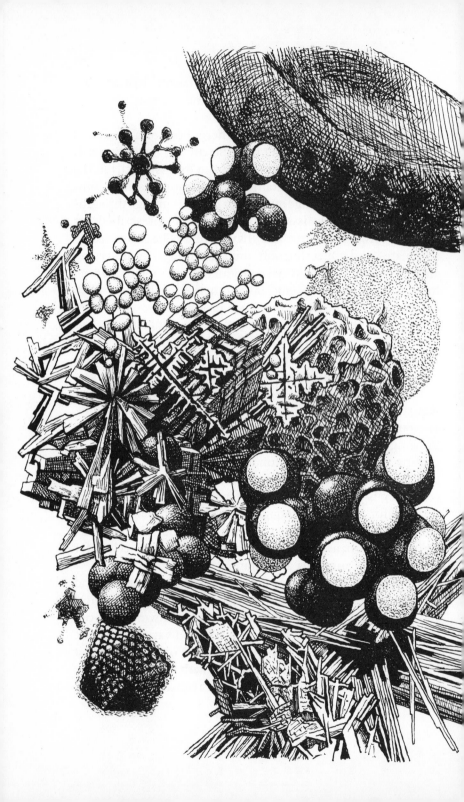

the white pulp succulently lining the coconut's outer hairy skin—is quite rich in sodium, as is the coconut milk itself, and this could account for the youthful bodies and long lives of many Polynesians, who use coconut in their everyday food. If you find fresh coconut indigestible, don't blame the coconut, blame your stomach. Get that digestive apparatus of yours in good working trim and you will digest coconut and any other fibrous, raw food with ease.

Many other foods could be listed for their sodium content, and most raw fruits and vegetables contain goodly quantities of it. As long as you don't overlook your ration from those high concentration sources—kelp and celery and dandelion and carrot and parsley—you should not lack natural sodium.

POTASSIUM

Potassium works in harness with sodium to help regulate body-fluid balance. Just as plant nutrients have to be taken through the soil to their roots by water transport, so human cells need body fluids circulating freely around them to interchange cell foods and cell wastes through membrane walls. Often a 'water tablet' containing potassium salts is used as a medical treatment for such fluid imbalances as hypertension, or fluid retention in tissues causing overweight problems, or even high blood pressure, which can upset fluid patterns. *Natural* correction of these conditions includes a diet containing such foods as celery, cucumber, lettuce, cabbage, cauliflower, tomato, watercress, sorrel, dandelion greens —what a French salad combination! If you wonder why combinations of foods have evolved traditionally to be used together, there is often a very good reason. The French salad would balance the bread and meat or game dishes, slowly cooked in their gravies and sauces, which often preceded it at the table, so that by the time the gastric juices at their full strength had begun to digest the grain and the animal protein there would be a potassium flood from the salad to move such heavier food through the body fluids and outwards into the bloodstream at the right speed. Without such a salad, a convivial French family might well bog down in a stupor of slow and incomplete digestion.

The primary site of potassium metabolism is in the liver, where glycogen is formed and stored. This is the substance that feeds muscles and ligaments and cartilage with dextrose —a sugar fuel—when muscle activity is needed. If your liver is healthy you store maximum reserves of glycogen and have good muscular energy and response whenever you need it. Here is another reason for the French salad: all that rough red country wine or lovingly matured special vintage tends to overload the liver if taken to excess. I'm not saying that a green salad can enable you to drink another glassful without damage, but it can help restore your liver function (which is now working hard on the wine), especially if such a salad has a good vegetable oil and garlic and lemon-juice dressing (vitamin F and vitamin C). The elasticity and tone of muscles depends mainly on potassium.

The biochemical reaction of potassium is alkaline, so it helps balance acid accumulations in the body. Potassium-rich foods should be eaten often by arthritic and rheumatic sufferers. Although the initial effect may be a 'stirring' one, movement and change of fluid balance causing *more* dis-comfort in the affected bones and joints, the end result is a good one because uric acid is flushed out and away from painful areas. Many arthritic folk say, 'I can't eat tomatoes, they really upset me; they're too acid.' This is the stirring effect that can lead an arthritic to believe tomatoes make his condition worse, not better. Tomatoes are a particularly rich source of potassium, and this mineral counterbalances their citric, mallic and oxalic acid content. Although on the kitchen cutting board they have an acid pH of about 4.25, this changes in the digestive processes to an alkaline pH 8.3, nothing for an arthritic to worry about.

Potassium is essential in the fluids between cells, the fluids that take it to and from the cells. Because it regulates muscle function it also helps the heart, a major muscle, and regulates the irritability or excitability of muscles, thus ensuring good tone and, after use, good relaxation patterns of muscle fibres.

A deficiency of potassium can lead to bad elimination of fluid wastes through the kidneys, and cause all kinds of diseases. An accumulation of unremoved rubbish builds up ideal conditions for infection, and can result not only in lethargy but in chronic major metabolic disorders. Have that salad at least once a day!

Sources of potassium (as well as tomatoes) are all the edible seaweeds (kelp, dulse, agar, Irish moss); legumes; dried fruits, particularly dried apricots and bananas; rice bran and wheat bran; wheatgerm, chick-peas and sesame seeds; and all dried beans have a high potassium content. That little-known vegetable, New Zealand spinach, is a rich source, and makes a welcome variation as a steamed green vegetable. Then there are radishes and beetroot, and (one of my favourite pre-packaged meals) the avocado. In winter time it is possible to get more heat and fuel energy from one avocado and two ripe bananas for lunch than you would get from a bowl of steaming hot soup.

Coconut meat is high in potassium, coconut milk high in sodium; so here is another of Nature's 'package' meals where one whole food contains a nutritional balance.

Parsley is so high in potassium that parsley tea is often recommended for rheumatic and arthritic and fluid-retaining patients as a simple home-corrective measure. Possibly the most concentrated in all minerals and vitamins of any food except kelp, parsley should be in or on your meals somewhere each day.

Sunflower seed is an excellent potassium source, too. Many men with minor fluid problems involving prostate gland enlargement have found relief by eating sunflower seeds regularly. Horseradish has probably for generations kept the English roast beef and Yorkshire pudding devotees from intestinal sogging. That small amount of horseradish relish on the roast beef would provide enough potassium to make some sort of digestion possible.

Fresh peaches are the best fruit-source of potassium. Serve them at the end of a heavy meal, glowing pinkish-green and ripe; or serve them as a meal alone on a steamy humid late-summer day. With a few grapes and a dob of yoghurt on top, a bowl of fresh peach-halves is refreshing and cooling.

If you feel dried-out and heavy and somehow sense that what you need is a good flush-out and cleansing of the system of built-up wastes, go for potassium-rich foods and feel the blocked tissues clear.

IRON

Iron is vital to the growth of any living organism. In an average-sized human body of about 70 kilograms there are approximately 3.5 grams of iron; and there are ten times more of this iron in the bloodstream than anywhere else. It is found in the red blood cells as haemoglobin, and its action in the body must be triggered by that trace of copper present, as well as by a certain amount of chlorophyll, the green colouring matter found in the leaves of plants and vegetables. Without this trace of copper, iron remains inactive and virtually useless, unable to go about its business of transmitting oxygen and allowing the tissues of the body to 'breathe'. If you haven't enough iron in your foodstuffs you may be afflicted by many ailments: repeated colds, influenza attacks, and inflammatory disease symptoms (any illnesses conveniently labelled '-itis', such as tonsillitis, conjunctivitis, hepatitis); and you may find that your body's ability to heal and to incinerate waste products is less than it should be.

Iron not only burns up a lot of garbage, it regenerates as well, transporting oxygen to every cell in the body. If you have a fever from some severe inflammatory attack, you need lots more iron in its natural forms to give strength to every body cell, to make the whole organism capable of fighting off the invading bacteria or viruses. For any injuries to soft tissues the body needs iron, for obvious reasons when bleeding or bruising has occurred either outwardly or inwardly. Iron is needed in producing the respiratory enzymes catalase and peroxidase, which control and co-ordinate respiratory function.

Females are much more likely to have iron prescribed for them than males. Women use about 15 to 30 milligrams of iron in each menstrual period, and this loss is sufficient—if not overcome by including high natural sources of iron in the diet—to produce symptoms of anaemia. Approximately 500 milligrams of iron are lost during childbirth, and this is when mothers should start munching away at parsley and watercress and strawberries, and all the other natural sources of iron. Young children and adolescents need more iron than average, and so do pregnant women to ensure that the foetal circulation is adequate without depleting their own body's iron reserves. If iron is found to be deficient in a man, it may be that some recent injury has produced blood loss and therefore loss of stored iron, or that a poor diet prevents him from assimilating properly the iron he does get. Blood loss always calls for extra iron. The bleeding may be slow or fast, internal or external, a nose-bleed, haemorrhoids bleeding spasmodically over a period of time, ulcerated areas in the gastro-intestinal tract leaking small but constant amounts of blood.

In the animal protein group, most of the free iron is found in organs, such as the brains, heart, and liver. The highest source of animal iron is found in the livers of cattle, and in this form it is sometimes prescribed when a low iron factor is observed from the patient's symptoms. Vegetarians must obtain iron from other sources, and there is an abundance of it in all the green, leafy vegetables, particularly in the darker leaves. Iron is also in high concentration in some seeds, particularly in the germ of the wheat. A good spoonful of wheatgerm sprinkled over your breakfast cereal or fruit will be almost enough for your daily requirement.

Iron works in harness with calcium, and most natural remedies for iron deficiency symptoms contain quantities of calcium, to ensure the most satisfactory absorption of whatever iron is given.

Kelp again heads the list—here as the highest readily available source of natural iron. What a complete and highly useful vegetable this is! It has retained all the heavy minerals as well as the light ones we have lost from our soils, and it returns these minerals to us from deep on the ocean floor. You get about 1 per cent of iron in any quantity of kelp you take as a food supplement, and you need only between 9 and 20 milligrams of iron each day to meet your body's whole requirement.

Natural unprocessed bran, either from rice or wheat, gives you plenty of iron and tones up your bowels as well. Pumpkin seeds, dried and fresh, are high in this mineral, and sesame seed, the perfectly proportioned grain, follows not far behind. Soya beans are exceedingly rich in it, as are most of the bean family, so they should figure in the diet of vegetarians, as should molasses, that old-fashioned, sticky, black mess we swallowed when young—at the instigation of our grandmothers, probably, who were well aware of its health benefits although perhaps unaware of why it had such good results. Oatmeal is a good iron food, and so are wholewheat and whole barley: you get a daily ration from your muesli or your porridge if that is what you prefer for breakfast. Egg yolks are OK too, the iron being of animal origin here. They are easily assimilated and can be used in many ways in a natural diet.

Buttermilk and yoghurt both contain iron. They are already partly processed towards digestion and therefore are good foods to include if your digestion is weak, or if you are recovering from some illness. Prunes are extremely rich in minerals, too, iron amongst them. Fresh young green peas straight from the pod you could call a gourmet's approach to getting some natural iron: their succulent, sweet taste adds liveliness to hot dishes or cold salads. Avocado, that other gourmet's delight, is a food with a perfectly balanced set of mineral components, iron being amongst the most important. It is digested very quickly and easily, and one or two avocados each day could keep you alive and well. They may be luxury items where you live, but just think: there is a whole meal for you wrapped up in one olive-green 'alligator' skin that takes you less than a minute to prepare and only a few minutes to eat. And I cannot talk about iron without including once again the leaves of the dandelion, in which every vital mineral needed by your body is present. In general, the darker the fruit, vegetable, or grain, the more iron it contains.

Iron burns up the accumulated toxic wastes in the body and eliminates them altogether, and natural iron cannot give you constipation. It takes synthetic iron to do this. If you study the list of foods rich in iron you will see that most of them have laxative properties. Such foods as dates and figs, molasses, prunes, raisins, sultanas, currants, and plums, and grapes, too—all are abundant in iron and often eaten to reduce constipation naturally and to prevent its recurrence. You will need no synthetic iron preparations if you learn which foods contain this mineral in abundance.

One food we have omitted so far, and it's always a controversial example, is the banana. There are more misconceptions about the banana than there are about potatoes. Bananas fresh and—if you can obtain them—bananas dried naturally are sources of iron that are available all the year round in most temperate climates and that are complete foods in themselves for everyone from the smallest child to the most senior of citizens. And one or two bananas will ensure that your daily ration of iron is catered for.

Iron is such a vital mineral in illness that we often forget its preventive value. An apple a day may or may not keep the doctor out of your street, but a few sprigs of parsley and a daily spoonful of kelp granules sprinkled over your evening meal can ensure that your doctor drives elsewhere! You could call iron the greatest of the fuel elements, providing heat and energy and the driving force that stops us being sedentary, ruminative creatures and gets us up and doing. Without sufficient oxygen a fire cannot burn, a tree cannot grow, and a human being cannot live; and without iron in the bloodstream of the human being oxygen could not be used in the first place. Soils need iron to oxygenate them; plants grow more prolifically and strongly with it, and reproduce better; and where there are deficiencies in other mineral elements a booster of natural iron can break the pattern and restore better function.

MAGNESIUM

Magnesium is the mineral we need most if our nervous system is not functioning as it should; and, like all the other minerals we have dealt with, it needs a partner, phosphorus, in order to react efficiently. Seventy-five per cent of the magnesium in our bodies is found in the bones; but its most important function is in regulating the white nerve fibres that control the central nervous system, thus ensuring that correct signals go along the intricate network of nerves and nerve plexuses for the correct function of muscles and organs. Magnesium also helps to regulate glandular function, which is closely related to the nervous system in many ways, for this central control gives impulses to glands as well as to other parts of the body. Magnesium is essential for health, and lack of it can cause anything from chronic irritability and exhaustion to mental retardation and mental illness when the deficiency is severe.

Magnesium is the necessary element when spasmodic contraction of muscles occurs, as in cramps, in muscles sore from unexpected over-use, and in chronic tension patterns when muscles contract involuntarily under stress; in fact magnesium is necessary whenever muscular contraction is damaging. Athletes all want their muscles to contract and tighten and harden and function well under specific stress impulses that they consciously maintain, but involuntary muscular contraction can cause pain by occluding nerves or pinching, so that the pain sets up a secondary contraction of the body as it attempts to escape from the pain itself. Even children born with spastic conditions considered to be quite severe have been treated with magnesium compounds with some degree of success. Magnesium, calcium, and phosphorus: these are the 'big three' minerals needed for modern living, to combat its speed and its stresses.

Magnesium plays a part in hardening the teeth, which makes it a modern-day mineral, a weapon against the tooth decay and degeneration we have come to accept as inevitable in our world of today. The glandular system of the body is one of the first to suffer from the stress of living as we do. Everything from sterility to hypothyroidism has been treated with magnesium, with positive results when the glandular dysfunction can be traced to a lack of it. It is alkaline in its reaction and so counteracts the acid inflammatory condition of nerve endings caused by stress. One of magnesium's most useful compounds for human metabolism is its phosphate, for in magnesium phosphate the two minerals necessary for happy, healthy nerves are both present. It can be slightly laxative in its action, and so helps to reduce the volume of waste products and to make their elimination easier.

One very important property of magnesium is its stimulatory action on enzyme function. As we have mentioned before, enzymes provide the basic difference between a living and a dead organism. If you want to walk around fully alive, magnesium is for you! Sometimes, if you feel half dead, this exhaustion can be attributed to insufficient magnesium and phosphorus in foodstuffs. To feel vital and alive, *electrically* alive, we need both these minerals. I say 'electrically' because our nervous system is in effect our lighting system. It lights us up. Without the necessary nervous impulses to keep every cell in our body alive, we should all grind to a stop. This electrical system of ours can become jangled or scrambled unless the necessary minerals are there to provide good communication links from one part of the body to another. It is not the task of this book to investigate microcellular electrical responses, fascinating as they are to me, but I can tell you that without magnesium and phosphorus there would be no light or life in us at all.

Those of you who enjoy a proportion of alcohol somewhere in your fuel intake, may like to understand just what it does to your nervous system. Do you get sleepy-drunk? If you do, you should understand what is happening inside you. The alcohol is depressing the functioning of your magnesium/ phosphorus team. This is why alcohol can give you that certain feeling of relaxation, and can in larger quantities relax you so much that you fall down ungracefully on the footpath or slide, more gracefully, underneath the table! Quite seriously, alcohol can so inhibit magnesium function that your muscles just can't tighten even if you want them to. In smaller quantities it can most certainly ease some of those frustrations and tensions that stop you enjoying yourself; but in excessive amounts it causes you to lose control not only of your muscles but of your central nervous system as well. The chief reason for this is the sudden or progressive inhibition of the function of magnesium in controlling your nervous system.

Neuralgia sufferers can benefit greatly from increased intake of magnesium. And the herb valerian is a gift of the plant kingdom to the nerve fibres of humans: it has a complete and perfect balance of magnesium phosphate and calcium phosphate, together with many other components.

For magnesium-rich foods I would like to find you a different candidate to head the list, but I'm aftaid we're stuck once again with our old friend kelp. What an incredible source of mineral elements this plant substance is! What a friend and benefactor to all of us who cannot lead an idyllic life of simple rustication! Wheat products are again high on the list—wheat bran and the germ of the wheat being exceedingly rich in magnesium. Most of the nut family contain abundant magnesium, in particular almonds and cashews, with Brazil nuts and walnuts following not far behind, and pistachio nuts and pecans only slightly lower on the list. Sesame seed confronts us again here, small and soft and completely bland to the system: it's no wonder that Ali Baba thought of sesame as a magic word to open to him the riches of his secret cave.

I shall take up arms in defence of one of my favourite salad vegetables here: the tomato. Tomatoes seem to have no lukewarm friends or acquaintances—you are either for 'em or agin' 'em. I have never found the tomato to produce any of the adverse reactions that are widely attributed to it. Its extremely high content of magnesium puts it near the top of the list as a salad vegetable. Spinach is a good source of magnesium too, and I cannot agree with any of the arguments against it. Lettuce, too, for its magnesium and many other virtues. If you can manage to grow your own baby lettuces, even if it's in a tub on your home-unit balcony or in a prune tin on your back porch, it is worth every minute of time and effort you spend doing it. Lettuce is one of the fastest dehydrating vegetables of them all, and should be picked and eaten while it is full of life.

We find the dandelion here too, its green leaves being saturated with magnesium as well as with so many other life-giving minerals, and watercress and cabbage and celery, too—and what a pleasant vegetable this is when it's fresh and full of life and still retains the high water content it had when it was growing. Don't ever buy celery that is flabby and flaccid: its nutritional value is less than half what it was when it was newly picked. Radishes, particularly the small round variety, are rich in magnesium, and they are the finest things you could want for your nervous system's conditioning. Parsley is here as everywhere else, and—garlic. Not only your nerves but your general health will benefit when garlic is in your diet.

There is more magnesium found in salad vegetables than in most other sources, but we must not forget the soya bean. Lecithin from soya beans is a mighty valuable source of magnesium and phosphorus, both in the daily diet and remedially for an overloaded nervous system. Potatoes cooked in their skins are high in magnesium content, and so is the common banana, especially when it is fully ripe and getting to that dark, squashy, sweet stage. Dried apricots and dates should be included too, as tasty nibbles when you're feeling peckish, or to renew nervous energy whenever you need it.

Magnesium is found in comparatively larger quantities in vegetables and fruits and some of the grains than are others of the mineral family. These foodstuffs should be eaten as preventive medicine, not only to renew our tired nervous systems but to prevent their getting tired in the first place. It's so simple to prepare a mixed varied salad of freshly picked greens; and it's such a health-giving culinary delight that we should surely have one on our menu every day.

CHLORINE

Large quantities of chlorine exist as chlorides in most foods, so we don't have to be so selective in choosing sources of it. The popular confusion of chlorine in the body with sodium chloride or common table salt has caused the first of several gross misunderstandings. Chlorine combines with sodium to act as a body cleanser, expelling waste matter, cleaning the blood, and tending to reduce fat or certain types of over-weight conditions in the process. But taking common salt is most certainly not the way to get these two valuable minerals into your body.

Let's do a little biology and biochemistry and anatomy, and find out why excess common salt in the diet can give rise to many overweight conditions, even resulting in oedema and congestive heart failure. Many of you have been advised by your doctor or naturopath to reduce or entirely eliminate salt in your diet when heart problems are present, or when obesity—a heart-stressing condition—is the problem. Aldosterone is the salt-retaining hormone secreted by the adrenal glands, the small pair of glands sitting atop your kidneys and sometimes known as the suprarenal glands. Any dysfunction or malfunction of the adrenal glands could cause retention of salt and therefore retention of fluid in body tissues.

What causes dysfunction of the adrenals? There are many causes, but one of the basic ones is an impeded flow of blood to the liver, the organ that regulates aldosterone balance. It follows, then, that if you treat the liver and its blood supply you will eliminate much of your fluid retention problem if it is coming from this combination of circumstances. I call it the yellow system—the liver, pancreas, bile duct, spleen, and bladder—and it is interesting to find that chlorine regulates most of the functions of this system. Chlorine is acid-forming in the body, but it stimulates enzyme activity as well as gastric secretion, and therefore the whole of the digestive tract. If you haven't enough natural chlorine in your body tissues you may have weak water-retention and decrease in body weight because of it. Deficiency of chlorine can also lead to liver problems, particularly under-activity of the liver, and to congestive disorders of many different types, such as swelling of feet and legs, lumps and cysts and fatty deposits, the congestion that goes with chronic sinus or bronchial problems, and even congestive heart disease.

People who pick up the salt-shaker and sprinkle before they have even tasted what is on the plate should stop and think what this is doing to the waistline. The food they are eating need not necessarily be the cause of their overweight problem—it could be the salt they are shovelling on top of it. Salt from vegetable sources does not have this effect of retaining fluid in the body tissues, and those who like a salty tang to their meals would be wiser to invest in a good vegetable salt.

If you give up salt entirely you will find that your taste buds become surprisingly reactivated, and you can really savour and enjoy nuances of flavour you never appreciated before because of the all-pervading taste of salt. Try gradually cutting down on your salt intake, even your vegetable salt addition, and see how you can once again discriminate between flavours in the way Nature intended. The taste buds of animals are so selective that the chemical responses produced in them by different foodstuffs determine whether they will or will not eat the food without any conscious choice taking place. The taste buds make the choice for them.

Tomato and celery head the list here, with lettuce not far behind, and kelp ever present. Spinach and cabbage and parsnips are rich in chlorine, as are turnips and horseradish. Whenever kidney malfunction is suspected, or any abnormal functioning in the yellow system, horseradish can be eaten with great benefit. Watercress has chlorine, too, and so has rhubarb. Some people say that the oxalic acid in rhubarb is harmful, pointing out that gallstones and kidney and bladder stones and gravel are composed mainly of calcium oxalates. But evidence in case histories of patients with stone and gravel problems has never in my experience showed an overloading of oxalic-acid-containing foods in the diet. It takes some malfunction or disorder in the organs themselves before oxalates can build up as rock-like evidence of the weakness in this portion of the metabolic process.

Eggplant is a good source of natural chlorine, and there are so many unusual, tasty ways of preparing it (even if you are not Italian or Greek) that you should have no difficulty in including eggplant dishes in the menu regularly when this magnificent vegetable is in season. Avocados contain chlorine too, and so does the sweet potato, that versatile vegetable that can be used either in the savoury section of the meal or whipped up into old-fashioned purees and puddings that have a sound nutritional basis. Asparagus, so salutary in its action on kidneys and bladder, contains chlorine, and so do dandelion greens.

Brussels sprouts in season are amongst my favourite vegetables and I steam them quickly with a dob of butter, (yes, butter, not margarine) to give colour and taste variation to winter vegetable hotpots. Unusually high on the list come the common banana and the pineapple. Both these fruits have drawbacks to a lot of people, one for its so-called fattening properties and the other for its so-called acid properties. Chives are chlorine-rich, and so are raisins, and some tropical fruits like guava, mango, breadfruit and watermelon. Figs are not what you would call saturated with chlorine, but they do come about the middle of the list, and so do sunflower seeds and peaches.

In speaking of foods that are rich in a particular mineral, I am not listing all the foods that contain it, but merely giving you a selection of the more common and available ones so that you will know a little more about their properties when you put them on your dinner table.

SILICON

Silicon is a mineral whose metabolic relationships and action have recently been investigated. It has been found to play an important role in preventive medicine, particularly in dietary control and prevention of further deterioration in arthritic conditions, as well as in many other body functions including our protective outer layer, the skin. After oxygen, silicon is the most abundant element in soil and sand, and is found mostly as its dioxide. It is essential to plant life, and appears to be most essential in the early days of the plant's growth: every gardener knows that seeds and seedlings will fare better and germinate in a more healthy, vital manner if they are started off in sand particles rather than in a garden loam. The crystalline structure of silicon is arrow-shaped, and this could have something to do with breaking up the outer shell of seeds so that the germ of life within can start to function.

In humans the action of silicon is complex, but its general activity is to preserve calcium metabolism from distortion or loss, therefore tending to prevent the formation of nodes and spurs and calcium deposits round joints, which are the obvious outward symptoms of advanced arthritis. The arrow-shaped crystals actually break up uric acid crystals round affected joints and bones, and aid greatly the reassimilation of such acid into the bloodstream and out through the excretory channels. If there is not sufficient silicon in the diet, arthritic sufferers (particularly those in advanced stages of the disease) are being deprived of a natural, simple method of arresting the deterioration processes and of actually restoring some measure of function to twisted limbs and joints. This is not to say that if you eat celery all day your arthritis will disappear in a week—far from it. It is only common sense and reason, however, to include as many silicon-rich foods as you can in your diet so that you can mitigate the crippling effects of the lack of silicon that would appear to have caused the condition in the first place.

Silicon has another important function: it has to be present in sufficient quantities to give us healthy nails and hair. Calcium we need as well, but without silicon the calcium cannot go about its work of strengthening fingernails and conditioning hair. Silicon's action on this outside layer of ours appears to be that of piercing 'holes', so that any unexcreted 'garbage' lying just underneath the skin in cells and tissues can be discharged by suppuration through the skin itself. In this day of allergy reactions it is a necessary mineral to remove sick and dead cells from the skin, thus lessening its susceptibility to the irritative agents that abound in our smoggy air and chemicalised environment. Silicon is prescribed to correct excessive sweating from head and feet, and excessive general body sweating; to promote more natural excretion rather than eliminating many body toxins through the skin by way of sweat glands. Excessive perspiration from any part of the body is often an indication that other excretory organs of kidneys and bowel are not working as efficiently as they might and that the skin is taking the burden of their work.

Silicon is also found in bones and various organs of the body, and in the nerve sheaths, the insulating material around the nerve fibres themselves: so you can see that your nervous system also demands silicon in a protective role.

Lettuce is the best of all the silicon-containing foods readily available to us. It has so many virtues, but this is one of its finest. So eat that enormous dark-green outer leaf of the lettuce when it's put flat on the plate underneath your mixed salad, knowing that if it's dark and coarse it is one of the outer leaves of the vegetable, and therefore much higher in its mineral content than the delicate inner heart leaves. Parsnips and asparagus come next, and they're followed by the army of dandelion greens marching again loaded with minerals and given to us freely and abundantly by Nature. Horseradish contains lots of silicon and so do spinach and cucumber, and also that food we don't need much excuse to eat—and can eat even more appreciatively now we know how chockful of minerals it is—the strawberry.

Sunflower seeds are the first amongst the grain seeds, and pumpkin is here too, the seeds containing about the same proportion of silicon as the flesh. Then we come to celery, with not only the perfect ratio of potassium and sodium but an abundant share of silicon as well. Fresh apricots are a good fruit source of the mineral, and so are tomatoes, carrots and turnips. Millet contains quite a high proportion of silicon for a grain, and it's preferred as a grain food by athletes the world over, for it builds strength without adding too many calories.

Fresh apples—not apples that have been in cold storage all the previous season—contain silicon, and so do most of our vegetable foods like cabbage and potato. Brown rice is pretty good too, and even lemons have some silicon, which is one of the lesser reasons why lemon is often an ingredient in skin-toning preparations.

Oats is a grain product that I firmly believe should be included every day somewhere in everyone's diet. It has so many valuable properties—structural, muscle-building, circulatory, digestive, eliminatory and tonic—that there are good reasons why it should be a staple in every diet. And it contains more silicon than any of the other foods I have mentioned. Oat-straw, the outer husk of the oats, which is usually winnowed away, contains the most silicon in the grain; so if you can obtain whole oats you are sure of getting the maximum dose of silicon available. Oat-straw tea is available from your health store to make a pleasant natural drink when added silicon is needed for any therapeutic reason.

I have a family history of arthritis and a predisposition to it; so foods high in silicon are among my favourite tastes and flavours. I have written elsewhere about instinctive food cravings. I need only say here that it's no wonder I am drawn to foods rich in silicon, for my body naturally prefers to live healthy and strong rather than get arthritis. Let me impress upon you that the treatment of arthritis is not a simple matter—far from it—but it is preventive medicine we are concerned with, as well as simple corrective procedures. If you have a history of arthritis-type conditions in your family tree, don't let this happen to you. Eat the preventive foods that will keep your body free from this affliction.

SULPHUR

Sulphur, in organic compounds, is found spread prolifically about in most foods, particularly in protein foods, which usually contain about 16 per cent nitrogen and 1 per cent sulphur. Unlike other minerals, sulphur is commercially available in its natural form (as an element) and can therefore be assimilated by the body when it is artificially introduced into foodstuffs such as dried fruits. If you have ever bought sun-dried apricots or prunes or any other naturally dried fruits you will know that they have a blackish-brown colour that looks rather unpleasant; but when they are soaked in water the original flavour and goodness are restored. Sulphur is added to many of the dried fruits to retain their natural colour, and I have not found it to be as harmful as many of the other food-preserving agents and artificial colouring compounds. Insulin is a sulphur compound, so it follows that diabetic patients should try to eat foods high in this mineral. Vitamin B_1 has also been found to contain sulphur: its use in the body is a complicated one of absorbing and cleansing by recycling waste products back into the bloodstream and out through the excretory organs rather than through the skin.

Sulphur is found in all body tissues and in haemoglobin in the blood, and it is needed for the formation of amino-acids and in the metabolism of proteins, too. Nature has again provided for us by ensuring that small quantities of sulphur are found in most protein foods, so that the metabolism can go ahead without hold-up. It has a cleansing and antiseptic action on the whole of the digestive tract. Some of you may have been forced to take sulphur and treacle or sulphur and molasses when you were young, and now you know why such an unpalatable mess was shoved down your throat: the sulphur and the iron did a good job of cleansing the blood-stream and the digestion and making you like new again.

One of the most common symptoms occurring in modern living is skin sensitivity arising from too high an intake of protein foods, which the body is struggling hard to digest but is finding beyond it. Even vegetable protein, such as that found in soya beans, can sometimes produce such symptoms if you get carried away and eat too much of it. Too much animal protein can, of course, do this too, and is much more likely to be the cause in countries where there is high protein intake from animal sources, together with lack of exercise and a faulty diet. Sulphur acts as an oxidising agent on the blood, and in the form of sodium sulphate it has a powerful equalising effect, and a stirring effect as well, on body fluids. The secretion of bile is improved, and therefore digestion; and toxic matter is prevented from accumulating in cells and tissues. If you have a skin condition that is not responding to silicon, try some sulphur-rich foods as well, for your skin irritation problem may be coming from a lack of this vital element.

The whole of the onion family is a veritable treasure store of sulphur. All its members—from common white or brown onions to leeks and shallots and spring onions, from chives and Welsh onions to the daddy of them all, garlic—are rich sources of available sulphur. Garlic is so high in sulphur that it will reabsorb and remove deep pockets of infection you may not even be aware of: they will steadily and slowly disappear as the sulphur 'broom' sweeps them back into the bloodstream and out.

Let's go back to our familiar list again: it's still watercress and brussels sprouts and horseradish; it's cabbage and it's spinach and, of course, it's kelp and radishes and cucumber and lettuce. Celery is back again, and asparagus and avocados, with tomatoes somewhat lower in the list. We have carrots and eggplant and turnip greens; we have grapefruit and pineapple and sweet corn; potatoes and dandelions are back too, and figs and a newcomer to add, Jerusalem artichokes. Soya beans, built as they are by Nature to be a balanced food, do contain sulphur, so that although an excess of soya beans in your diet can produce various symptoms of protein allergy owing to dryness of the bowel, the modicum of sulphur contained therein makes this unlikely if you are sensible about how much soya bean you have every day. Watermelons and strawberries and apples and oranges; cherries and pumpkin; raisins and mushrooms...down we go again through all the familiar foods, finding sulphur in them too.

It is often the case that vegetables with a rather bitter

flavour, such as brussels sprouts and horseradish, and even cabbage and turnip and cauliflower, are the highest in sulphur. But you can almost smell the stuff sizzling away in every vegetable calling itself a member of the onion family. In pure garlic oil, extracted by pressure from the cloves, the sulphur content can be as high as 80 per cent. It's no wonder garlic does such a job of cleansing and antibacterial warfare. Its only drawback is that we smell sulphurous while it's doing it!

IODINE

Iodine is a vital element, specifically for the thyroid gland. Since the thyroid controls indirectly or directly every metabolic process, its health and efficient function are exceedingly important to the body as a whole. If you live up to 50 kilometres from the seashore it is odds on that you are getting sufficient iodine as onshore winds blow iodine-laden salt over you and over the soil around you. But if you live much farther away from the sea and do not have foods rich in iodine in your diet, there may be a tendency in that area for thyroid imbalance to occur in the population in general. There are many areas where iodine is virtually unavailable naturally, so iodine supplements or foods rich in it must be taken not only to prevent severe disease but to maintain even average health. This is where kelp really shines—1.5 per cent of it (by weight) is organic iodine. It's an enormous proportion when we find that the first garden vegetable on the list, green turnip tops, contains only 0.0007 per cent. Perhaps our need for iodine comes from our primitive origins, which we are told were in the seas, when our body metabolism was tuned to absorption of iodine. Perhaps you could call kelp the transitional food, the last link with our marine past.

All the foods rich in sulphur and in silicon turn up here again, but with very much lower concentrations of iodine. Indeed, only minute amounts of this element are necessary unless there are symptoms pointing to a deficiency. The thyroid gland increases the oxidation processes in the body, and if its balanced function is disturbed, fluctuating patterns occur that can be distressing to the patient even if they do not cause severe illness. Correct thyroid activity is necessary in the oxidation of fats and proteins, and incomplete process- ing can cause the typical hypothyroid pattern of sluggishness and slowness as the body is loaded down with partly digested food. Kelp has a unique property in that it is a balancing agent, useful in both under- or over-activity of the thyroid gland. It regulates thyroxin no matter which way the picture goes. Even if you forgot all the other iodine-rich foods and ate only a teaspoonful of powdered or granulated kelp each day, you would ensure an average balanced state of this vital controlling gland.

Thyroid activity controls not only metabolic processes but other glands indirectly through hormonal activity, so it is important in maintaining the endocrine system in a state of balance and healthy function.

BROMINE

Bromine is an interesting mineral that has been found to be present constantly in the bloodstream. Its concentration varies under direct influence from the pituitary gland, the conductor of the whole glandular orchestra. In certain states of mental depression the bromine content of the blood has been found to be approximately one-half normal until the mental or emotional picture is corrected. This fluctuating pattern has also been suspected of causing pre-menstrual tension, that depressive and often tearful and emotional state affecting many women. Research is now showing that these depressed states relate directly to the bromine concentration in the pituitary gland. Even the fluctuating emotional patterns often associated with the menopause are now being traced to the bromine levels in the pituitary gland and the degree to which bromine is released, or not released, into the bloodstream to preserve emotional stability.

We might try to treat menopausal depression and premenstrual tension by a rapid intake of bromine-rich foods, and we have a surprising candidate here for top honours—watermelon. The melon fruits in general, such as rockmelon, cantaloup and honeydew, are all good rich sources of bromine, and countries where these melons are staple foods in the diet are countries with emotionally stable populations. That's a sweeping statement; but just think of the Polynesians whose diet includes so many of the melon fruits and who must have been amongst the happiest people when they lived in their natural state. Cucumber and celery rate with melons as foods containing high bromine levels, and so do asparagus and tomato and lettuce, followed by mushrooms and carrots and parsnips—all the same old goodies in slightly different order but still there. Garlic rates high here too, and so do millet and rye in their wholegrain form. Peaches are good bromine fruits, and so are apples, and the onion tails along somewhere near the end of the list. In both men and women the bromine content of body tissues starts to decrease from middle age, and in old age—say at seventy-five years onwards—hardly any bromine can be detected at all. If you wish to preserve a good emotional balance to keep you biologically younger than your chronological age, it would be an idea to consume melons whenever they are available.

TRACE MINERALS

The parts played by the so-called trace minerals—aluminium and tin, arsenic in minute amounts, nickel found in the pancreas, and mercury in the liver—are not yet fully understood. Is it only accidental that silver has been found in the tonsils and the thyroid gland, or does it play some delicate but necessary part in the overall health picture of these organs? Most of the trace minerals seem to appear in the glandular system, and whether this is significant or not has yet to be discovered. There may well be minute traces of all sorts of strange compounds and unknown elements that contribute to the total picture of life and health we all wish to attain. For there is no reason to suppose that everything is now known about the everyday workings and structure of the human organism. There may be whole new worlds to conquer not only in outer space but in inner space!

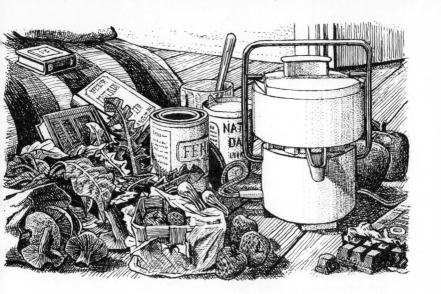

3

Instinctive Eating

When a woman seven months pregnant has a sudden craving for strawberries with mushroom sauce at two o'clock in the morning, gratify her irrational yearning if you can! Her instincts, surer than reason and logic, are prodding her into providing an immediate need for the unborn child—a massive dose of folic acid, an anti-abortion vitamin. For the foetus to remain attached by the placenta to the uterine wall, drawing its nourishment from the mother's body, it must have adequate folic acid 'glue'. Women with a history of miscarriages during the early months of pregnancy have been treated with folic acid and have produced healthy full-term babies. But why not supply folic acid naturally? Eat strawberries, mushrooms, lettuce, soya beans, all high in this vitamin, sometimes called vitamin M.

During a bout of flu some years ago I could eat nothing

and could drink only water for the first few days of high temperature, profuse sweating and convulsive shivering. Then I woke from my first real sleep for days with an overwhelming desire for pickles. I raided the fridge and sipped the juices from jars of pickled walnuts, cucumbers, and red cabbage. During the next few hours I felt a distinct change for the better. It was not until some years later that I read in an American medical journal of experimental work on the control of virus-type infections, using organic acids, in particular citric, oxalic and mallic acids. These naturally occurring acids were found to inhibit the growth and activity of the virus in the body cells without harming the cells themselves: and I realised then that my instincts had told me what my body needed.

In the short term, instinctive cravings for certain foods are almost always beneficial for the person concerned. But never confuse the artificial craving of the alcoholic for more and more alcohol with a natural, biological body signal: it is only a conditioned response to the body's and the mind's stress patterns—an escape, in other words, and a different thing altogether from a simple craving for sweets or cake, say. The housewife who nibbles compulsively and is seriously overweight is not satisfying a biochemical body need, only alleviating boredom or unhappiness by a constant occupational replacement—eating. A true acute nutritional need was recognised in wartime by navy mess orderlies, whose steaming cups of cocoa for those on duty gave immediate warmth, raised energy levels, and supplied a booster dose of phosphorus to help concentration. The balance of minerals in the cocoa bean is just right for providing peak levels of efficiency over short periods. It contains a stimulant for heart and circulation, raising the blood pressure and the body temperature. It follows, of course, that people with high blood pressure should not drink cocoa.

Those of us who get a sudden message from our internal computer saying 'chocolate', who buy a block and eat the whole lot in a matter of minutes, then never touch another piece for months or even years, are responding to a biochemical signal calling for an immediate increase in blood pressure, energy, body temperature, and nervous strength. This is no excuse for those who constantly eat chocolate—with a variety of unpleasant consequences. The clue to genuine instinctive biochemical impulses is that they don't come often and they don't repeat themselves after the immediate physiological needs have been satisfied. The demand for more of some favourite food that brings pleasant responses from the taste buds is different. The original signal comes from the palate cheering and asking for more, not the chemical computer busily adjusting and maintaining the body's equilibrium. The trick, of course, is to know which signal is which. These food cravings can be suppressed, controlled or ignored consciously and deliberately for many different reasons.

If you want to live as naturally as possible, always look at Nature and learn from her. A dog that is sick will nose about in grass clumps until it finds the appropriate remedy. Often it is couch grass, which the dog knows instinctively is what its body needs. But have you ever tried to make a well puppy-dog eat couch grass? It will sniff, turn up its nose and go elsewhere. When a wild animal is ill, the first thing it does is to stop and lie down. If only humankind had enough instinctive sense to continue doing as their animal ancestors used to do! A man who goes into the office when his sinuses are choked and aching, his head is congested and heavy, and his throat is raw, may be harvesting financial rewards, but he is overloading his body's capacity and undermining his future health. The instinctive need of any form of life when it is out of balance or equilibrium is rest. You could call this Nature's answer to illness: 'All systems *stop*'!

This brings us logically now to fasting. Animals fast as long as they need to—they go without food and sometimes without drink until their body control system tells them they can resume their normal nutritional habits. I remember a very enjoyable fast I did one Easter time when my family were away. I had no calls on my time, and four clear, sunny, beautiful days to do absolutely nothing. I did my own brand of fasting, which consisted of juicing three or four apples with two leaves of comfrey three times daily and drinking the thick green liquid immediately. In between times I brewed a cup of strong fenugreek tea to cleanse out toxic matter through the skin. I lay as bare as possible in the sunshine, soaking up its warmth and revitalising strength, and at the end of the four days felt completely renewed, cleansed and ready for the fray again. Guess what I ended my fast with? I bought the largest, juiciest, fattest piece of rump steak in town! My body's frantic signals told me it was now clean enough and needed rebuilding protein. I eat very little meat, but when I get such a clear, insistent message I follow it absolutely. Some of my natural-living friends recoil in horror when I tell them this story. I answer their disapproval very simply. 'That was what my body needed,' I tell them, 'and it knows better than I do what it wants and in what shape and form it will have it.'

Fasting produces swift incineration processes in the tissues, literally burning up and throwing out accumulated waste residues. If these waste materials are not removed, they create weak areas in the body where illness will settle when it comes: it's like carrying round half a dozen or so full garbage cans inside you for months, or even years. Although a healthy body is built to dispose of its own garbage efficiently and completely, it is sad to realise that I have never known— and I bet you haven't either—a completely healthy person. A short, sensible fast, with a few selected fruit juices or herbs, concentrates all the body's energy on breaking down rather than building up. A brisk spring-cleaning takes place in a short time.

Some people believe that a fast works more efficiently if an enema is taken during the fasting. Again I turn to Nature for her decision: animals don't have enemas. I do believe, however, that some form of natural bowel-cleansing agent should be taken for about a week or so before fasting. There is one particular herb, slippery elm bark, that is ideal. Slippery elm bark comes from a tree and is usually available in the form of a powder or tablets. It has a unique action on the whole of the alimentary system, lining every passageway from the throat and oesophagus through the stomach and intestines and the bowel itself. It lines, lubricates, heals and soothes any irritable or irritated spots anywhere in this system. It contains large amounts of natural calcium—that vital element for complete digestion of foods—thereby taking the weight off the digestive system as well, and ensuring that all waste matter is eliminated by a happy, healthy, soothed bowel. Slippery elm will stay in the body for approximately thirty hours, so a small dose each day for several days before your fast will ensure the maximum benefit from it.

When you get the feeling that your body is dirty, choked, clogged, heavy, and you decide to fast for a few days or longer, go onto your slippery elm conditioner first. Take a heaped tablespoon of the powder each day with either a mashed banana or mixed with a little honey, or make it into a paste with warm water then add to a glass of goat's milk, skim milk if you like it, or soya compound. If you prefer to take tablets, these are available from your health store too, with the dosage clearly marked.

Another way to cleanse and clear the bowel before fasting is to eat natural, unprocessed bran, the stuff we used to feed to chooks. This is one of the best intestinal brooms, sweeping out débris and giving tone to the bowel in the process. Start taking bran sprinkled on your morning muesli, on stewed or fresh fruit, with wheatgerm, any way possible really, because it is tasty and blends well with other cereal flavours. A good heaped tablespoon of bran once or even twice daily will start the elimination process and clear the bowel completely. Natural bran is recommended by the medical profession too. It is used as a dietary supplement for patients with diverticulitis, for it not only clears and strengthens the bowel but tones up its muscular action as well. Naturopaths have been recommending natural bran as a treatment for diverticulitis for a long time, for we know its action is safe, strengthening and efficient. At first you may have a bout or two of what appears to be diarrhoea, but it is certainly not a bad thing. This is only a sign that small pockets of putrid waste-matter in the bowel are being emptied and cleansed. It's like giving the back porch a good hose-down. Don't eat natural bran only as a preparation for fasting. It is something we all used to eat once and could all eat again with great benefit. Roughage and raw grain foods have a very toning effect on the bowel as well as the mechanical one of literally sweeping it out. Regard natural bran as preventive medicine—the ideal way to good health.

Short fasts are generally less arduous and more inviting and therefore easier. A fast of longer than four to seven days should not be undertaken without supervision by a trained naturopath or nutritionist, or someone who knows what he's doing with human metabolism. If you want to live on water and nothing else for a week, good luck to you—you will certainly feel different at the end of that time; but make it no longer than one week, especially if it is your first fast. A three- to four-day fast is always best to start with. Take it slowly—until you experience its benefits gradually, step by step, learning as you go. Some of my young students get so enthusiastic once the field of natural health is laid out there in front of them that they rush in headlong, determined to be super men and women overnight. Like all other natural processes, health comes in a slow, gentle, cumulative way. Don't go off into the wilderness with your boon companions determined to gaze at your navel and fast until you can fast no longer; you may become so weakened as to be in a dangerous physical state, even to lose consciousness, or you'll become dehydrated, miserable, and disenchanted. Extremes of any kind throw the whole organism out of Nature's balance. If you wish to fast only on water, this is fine and can be quite satisfactory. But if you wish to benefit one area of the body in particular (kidneys, stomach, liver, the muscular system, your circulation) you can fast on different fruit juices, or herbs juiced or fresh, which you know will not only cleanse but strengthen and renew that area. If your kidneys are not functioning as they should, forget trying to pinpoint what is the trouble: just fast on a juice and a few herbs to tone, strengthen, renew and restore function to those organs. A healthy pair of kidneys will repel any attack from any cause whatsoever. This is the whole basis of natural health and the instinctive patterns found in animals and in all other forms of life.

The strong can survive any attack. Strong kidneys, functioning as they should, filtering wastes as they were designed to do, will never be harmed by bacterial viruses or suffer from structural defects. This may sound revolutionary if you have been conditioned to think of illness as being caused by germs. Health is the natural state of all life: the unhealthy or weaker organisms just do not survive. So join the survival of the fittest, with all your body functions at their peak levels of efficiency. Natural medicine is always aimed at restoring the original state of good health by renewing the strength and function of whichever part of the body is under attack. When flu is going around, you have been taught that you may 'catch it'. Try to think of it this way. The flu is *always* around. You carry about with you in your body constantly a large number of bacteria, viruses, bacilli and assorted harmful or possibly harmful organisms. You can carry these organisms about for many years without any harm to you if your body is so healthy that they cannot grow, or propagate or destroy. But if they find an area in your body that is not strong and healthy, there they will focus, gather and eventually attack—with everything from a cold in the nose to cancer. Natural health measures are aimed at keeping the body's vitality and strength at such high levels that the assaults of illness cannot possibly make any progress.

Let's talk about the kidneys again. If you want to fast to increase the strength and function of your kidneys, try apple juice as your basic liquid intake together with, each day, a few sprigs of parsley and a very tiny mouthful of celery. Apple juice is almost neutral, neither very acid nor very alkaline, it is easy to digest, and it contains a large proportion of potassium, the element most needed and most lacking in the body if your kidneys are under-functioning. Parsley, one of the strongest and most powerful chemical combinations in the whole of the herb kingdom, contains a perfect balance of the sodium and potassium found in healthy kidneys. A small mouthful of celery (and make it a small one or you won't truly feel you are fasting) does likewise, adding traces of silicon and calcium and presenting the kidneys with a chemical picture identical with that of their own health. It sounds too simple perhaps, but health is simple.

If you're looking a bit green about the gills, the whites of your eyes are a dirty yellow, the skin under your eyes has a blackish, dead look, and you have soreness or pain or a heavy feeling under your right ribs, it is quite possible that your liver is not performing as it should. If you want to fast to improve the state of your liver, use dandelion coffee as your basic liquid intake, and chew each day a few fresh leaves of the common or garden dandelion, making sure you know which is a dandelion and which is not, and preferably not picking your dandelion leaves from round the base of telegraph poles. Too simple again? Not at all. Dandelions are a herbalist's dream, containing every element needed not only by the liver but by the whole body. They also contain choline, a vitamin that helps to control degeneration processes in the liver from age, from abuse such as alcohol, from stimulants such as too much black coffee, and from cirrhosis, a diseased condition in which liver tissue is replaced by hardened, dead scar tissue. There are many different treatments that can strengthen a weak liver, some of them very complicated. Why bother making life difficult when the simple dandelion can do the total job?

If your skin is dry, scaly, reptilian, and you look ten years older than your real age, this can have a frightfully demoralising effect, particularly if you are a female. A good fast programme for you would be cup after cup each day of fenugreek, comfrey tablets or, better yet, fresh comfrey leaves. Fenugreek tea contains vitamin A in the correct balance with vitamin D, the ideal combination for skin nutrition. It is also a diaphoretic agent—it can produce copious perspiration from every pore. Impurities just below the surface of the skin, sitting in the pores and follicles, accumulating in blackheads, pustules, pimples, and in some cases acne as well, are literally floated out in heavy perspiration. If the other eliminatory channels of your body—the kidneys, the bladder, the bowel—are not doing their proper job, your skin (often called the third lung) must bear some of the work. It covers the biggest area of any organ of your body—it can do a lot of eliminating! One friend of mine with chronically overloaded kidneys, because of a shocking diet that she refuses point-blank to change, can sometimes be talked into drinking fenugreek tea, and when she does so her perspiration smells like curry. The first time this happened she rang me in a terrible state saying, 'What have you done to me—I stink!' 'Good,' I said. 'That's one garbage can you don't have inside you any more.' I explained it all to her, and now she doesn't mind the consequences because she knows what is happening. She closes her doors on a Friday night, drinks fenugreek tea—two, three, sometimes four cups daily—and refuses to see a soul until Monday morning, by which time she smells like a rose.

It's no wonder the elimination produced by fenugreek smells like curry. It is a spice used in curry pastes and mixtures. Its hard little seeds, yellowish in colour, can be bought from your health store just as they came from the plant. You can also buy it ground to a fine powder, but the whole seeds retain more freshness. Grind them as you need them or soak them for 10 to 15 minutes in a little water before making your tea or adding them to a dish. The comfrey tablets or fresh comfrey leaves that you nibble as part of your fast programme contain two miraculous agents for skin. The first is one of the highest concentrations of vegetable calcium available and the second is a substance called allantoin, which speeds up the growth-rate of new skin cells. When you have finished your fast continue with the comfrey. Comfrey is the middle-aged lady's friend, the young lady's insurance policy, and the elderly lady's last resort. If you're ever going to look like the Queen of Sheba, comfrey can help you do it!

Here's a simple fast for sufferers from respiratory complaints. Drink fresh lemon juice or bought lemon juice with as little preservative added as possible, add a little honey if you can't stand its sour-bitter taste and chew a teaspoonful a day of aniseed seeds. Lemon juice cuts loose the phlegm and mucus adhering to the membranes of lungs, throat, nose and indeed the entire respiratory system. It contracts and tones up the soft membranes lining all these areas, preventing further mucous secretion, loosening and expelling the waste matter from the body. It helps the breathing, reducing the load on lungs full of soggy goo, and allows fresh oxygen to reach deep into the lung tissues, rejuvenating and stimulating their efficiency. As you will know if you like the flavour, aniseed is not at all difficult or unpleasant to take. Aniseed has an interesting property, too: it can vaporise mucus, loosening it and causing it to disintegrate so that the eliminatory processes can remove it through the bloodstream far more easily than you can by coughing, sneezing or blowing the nose. Fennel seeds can do the same thing, and can boost the action along with their high mineral content, particularly of iron and sulphur.

Fasting means different things to different people with

different bodies in different states of health. One cannot give a blanket decision, cannot say that fasting is good for you or that it is not good for you, because the circumstances vary and every one of us is different—thank the Lord!

I would never advise an arthritic patient to fast. There are many practitioners in my own field who disagree with me on this point, but I feel arthritis to be a particularly complicated, detailed, involved, and completely individual disease state. Arthritic patients suffer. They suffer inwardly as well as outwardly, because if they were not the type of person they are, if they did not suppress their woes, their wrongs, their stresses, and their frustrations, they would not have arthritis in the first place. That's a leading statement, and one that has produced a lot of controversy; but I firmly believe it is true. I would first treat the *person* rather than the disease alone, try to remove the stress patterns, try to rebalance the outlook. But the complete treatment of such a serious and destructive state of ill-health is outside the scope of this book.

There are simple straightforward fasts for flatulence and indigestion, perhaps caused by over-eating. You can go on a short four- or five-day fast chewing peppermint leaves and drinking grape juice—either light or dark, whichever appeals to you most in flavour. Peppermint, as you know from having sucked indigestion tablets, is always an ingredient in these remedies. It was used by the ancient Romans to overcome the indigestion from their three- and four-day feasts, and it worked just as well then as when we give our guests an after-dinner mint at the end of a long, sumptuous, special-occasion dinner. And if every dinner is a large, full, indigestible one—particularly at the end of a long, hard, stressful day—the stomach is going to complain loudly at having to work very hard while the rest of the body goes to sleep. No sooner do you lay your head on the pillow than the indigestion becomes unbearable. Your fast on grape juice and peppermint leaves (and nothing could be more refreshing and delightful) will give your overloaded, hardworked, protesting stomach a rest and allow it to sleep also. Grape juice contains several im-portant digestive acids, pectin, and other agents that aid, speed and control the rate of food absorption and digestion; and it is high in all the minerals, including trace minerals, needed for basic metabolism. A tired stomach, overloaded and busily trying to pass on to the bowel food that it cannot handle, will gratefully relax to do a more efficient job next time.

It is not always advisable to use orange juice as fluid during fasting. Although the three main citrus fruits—orange, lemon and grapefruit—are acid in reaction out of the body, lemon, and to a certain extent grapefruit, changes chemically as soon as it comes in contact with body fluids. It then has an alkalising action. Orange juice, however, does not change so dramati-cally or so beneficially. It is undoubtedly high in vitamin C content, but I feel it is grossly overrated as a source of this vitamin so essential to maintain body health and immunity to disease. There is nothing wrong with drinking small, medium or large quantities of orange juice, but for fasting there are better juices to try.

If you enjoy the feeling of lightness, strength and vitality after your fast is ended, make it a regular experience several times a year or more often if you wish. However, if you find after your fast that you feel no different, no better, and are disappointed with the results, it means that your body has been working so hard for so long with the wrong sort of fuel and the wrong sort of rest and recovery patterns that it will take much more positive, prolonged treatment to eradicate the cause of the problem.

Fast with a friend if you have no will-power. Each can encourage the other when the first pangs of hunger strike.

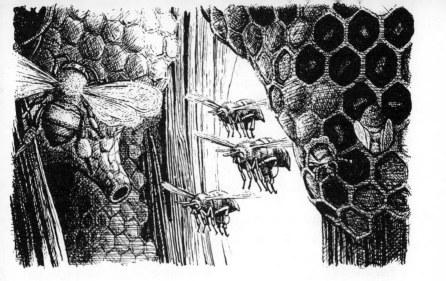

4

Good, Bad,
and Indifferent Food

It would amaze you to hear how many mothers like to 'fill the family up', and this is exactly what they do, until their poor sons and daughters and husbands succumb to some form of illness. One man's capacity is another man's overloading; but in general our stomachs can hold and absorb a certain amount of food only, and the surplus will remain in tissues and bloodstream and organs and muscles and nerves as an overload of useless garbage. It's not the quantity we eat that makes us well nourished: it's the quality of the food and the amount of nutriment it contains. You can lunch on a glass of apricot juice, with perhaps a touch of lemon juice to ginger it up, stirring in a tablespoon of wheatgerm and a teaspoon or two of yeast, munching a few sticks of celery and a couple of fresh carrots, and you will be sufficiently well nourished for the remainder of the afternoon. On the other hand, you may eat two meat pies with tomato sauce and two vanilla slices and a bottle of Coke and perhaps a cream bun and be utterly undernourished and hungry again by mid-afternoon. That sudden feeling of tiredness, those early-afternoon yawns, that wish to curl up in a corner and sleep, may mean that you had the wrong sort of lunch, that your body is over-occupied in digesting it, and becoming tired in the process.

If you make a habit of having no more than a cigarette and a cup of coffee before you rush off to work, you are building up a destructive cycle that will rapidly ruin your health. Perhaps you had a very large meal the previous evening, then stayed up quite late; and when you did go to bed you were not only tired but overtired, partly from digesting and partly from overworking or overplaying; then in the morning you were not sufficiently rested, you were not hungry, and facing the day seemed an intolerable burden. By mid-morning your spirits would be flagging, and you would be vaguely hungry, but you wouldn't really want to eat: you would be suffering a subclinical attack of malnutrition. By lunchtime you would be so hungry (your body so much in need of nourishment) that you would eat a luncheon of pies and cream buns and Coke in an effort to give yourself as much fuel as possible to get you through the afternoon. The tiredness would creep up around half past two to three, and by the time you got home for your evening meal you would be either so tired you'd not want to eat or so craving for nourishment that you would eat an enormous meal of meat and potatoes and other vegetables and bread, with a large sweet to follow and several cups of coffee—not to mention the alcohol before and after. And then you would wonder why your stomach was complaining so bitterly that you could not sleep. No wonder it's called a rat-race! With this sort of dietary pattern, you are endlessly running round that circle at top speed and getting absolutely nowhere.

One of the good things about good food is that you don't

have to eat enormous quantities of it, so that your digestive apparatus is not overloaded with unnecessary work and can absorb every bit of it. You may start by feeling hungry for a while if you suddenly reduce your intake and raise the quality level of your food, but after a week or two you will find that your stomach has contracted to a much smaller size, that its muscle tone is better and you do not have a nasty bulge below your waistline. You feel more energetic and somehow lighter —this is not surprising because you have lightened the load of fuel you are carrying. You will also find that mentally some of the cobwebs have blown away, some of the jungle has cleared as if by magic and you can see your way through it all.

It is difficult to classify a food as definitely good or bad for all of us. If the eating of fish or meat is an ethical taboo, it is obvious that good food is going to mean something different to you from what it means to the majority of meat-eating people. Individual tastes set the standards; but there are many foods that are undeniably good and nourishing, that can be absorbed to a greater or lesser degree by all of us, and that benefit our bodies in every way. These, naturally, are the ones we should aim to eat as often as possible; but it's a sad fact that 'civilised' living seems to compel us to rush through our day as 'efficiently' as possible, and we are tempted to buy prepared or ready-to-eat foods to save time—time we may later overspend in doctors' waiting-rooms.

There is no divine decree that says, 'Thou shalt eat three meals a day.' The digestion time for food varies with each one of us, but two to three hours is an average general diges-tion time for an average meal. You could suddenly feel hungry at ten o'clock in the morning if you had your break-fast a little before eight, and it is only custom and convention that says you must wait so many hours more before you have another meal. There is no reason why you shouldn't eat the right sort of food at ten or ten thirty to sustain you for another two to three hours. At the morning-tea break in the office, you could eat an apple and a small wedge of goat's cheese, or a tiny carton of cottage cheese and a little packet of nuts and raisins, and have a rosehip tea made from a tea-bag. You could then be the only one in the office—I'd stake my white coat on it—who would be feeling alert and vital at lunchtime and after lunchtime and well into the long afternoon. Some of us know perfectly well what we should eat, but are afraid of being laughed at as the odd-man-out. If you happen to be the only person in the office eating raw carrots with a slab of home-baked bread for your lunch and drinking peppermint tea in mid-afternoon, then you can regard yourself as the only sensible one present. If, when your energy requirements are greatest, when you need concentration and alertness, when your stomach plainly says 'I'm hungry', you can eat the good foods I'm going to discuss (the ones that seem appropriate to you), then you will have found a preventive medicine basis on which to build your own good-health pattern.

HONEY

I wondered which food was most appropriate to begin with in the short list I shall give of good foods. There are many that have claims to top position, but honey happens to be a favourite food of mine and one about which there are many misconceptions. To my mind, honey is one of the gifts of the gods, a food in its most concentrated and purest form, un-adulterated, unprocessed, manufactured only by the bees and the flowers, a food that can be assimilated by all of us in health and in illness, too.

Honey is a supreme natural food. Every part of its simple structure can be assimilated and in use in your body tissues within one hour. You can forget the obvious advantages of raw sugar, or even black sugar with its minerals, if you have a jar of honey in your office drawer or your kitchen cupboard and use this as your all-purpose sweetener. It can give you safe, fast energy. Any time when you feel your vital forces are depleted and you must press on, make yourself a pot of herb tea sweetened with honey, or take a tablespoon of honey in warm water. There are many claims made against honey: some say it rots the teeth, others say it's fattening, still others say it's too high in sugar content. I would say that all of them are wrong. The body assimilates any natural food only in the quantities it needs, throwing away any remainder; and it is impossible for your body to retain any excess honey with adverse effects. If your family has an urge for rice pudding, you can satisfy even this and still give them good food, using brown rice and honey and egg yolks and a little vanilla-bean flavouring, and goat's milk if you can manage it, or cow's milk if you really can't, or soy milk—best of all—from your health store. You can eat a goodly sized portion of the steaming, fluffy pudding without doing harm to yourself, especially if you sprinkle a little nutmeg and cinnamon on the top to aid its digestion, and a few raisins and sultanas to keep your bowels happy. If you use honey as your general sweetener you will get natural energy, direct from the sunshine and the flowers, in the shortest time.

FRUITS AND VEGETABLES

It goes without saying that fruits and vegetables are on our good food list, since they come to us (or should do) as Nature provided them. If you grow your own fruit and vegetables you can say with certainty that they are good for you; but if you are forced to buy your fruit and vegetables in shops this is not always true. The freshness of a good food is one of its virtues: it must be fresh from where it grew, and straight into your mouth in the shortest possible time. Fruits and vegetables have been covered fairly thoroughly in the chapters on vitamins and minerals, but I would reiterate that a fruit or a vegetable is only as good as its freshness. The organically grown unsprayed apples I ate in my friend's orchard at Bathurst remain one of the taste highlights of my life. When you can pick a fruit straight from the tree and eat it two seconds later you are getting food that is still 'living' with its vitamins and minerals intact. A good food must have as much life and vitality in it as possible. You know how a hot day can affect the appearance, the taste and the keeping quality of your greengrocer's merchandise: bought in the steamy hours of the morning, the fruit and vegetables are almost without life when you bring them to the table in the evening. Any living organism slows down to the point of death without its moisture quota. Living cells are compatible with other living cells and can revitalise with living energy.

There are many books on how to grow vegetables, even in the tiniest containers on your home-unit balcony or your kitchen window-sill. There is no excuse for you to say, 'I have no garden to grow my own.' Even growing some of your own—a few plants of this and that—is a positive step towards having living food. A small planting of carrots in a perforated plastic bucket; two or three lettuce seedlings in another smallish bucket; decorative pots full of parsley and chives and sage and thyme—these can fit into the tiniest area and can be easily looked after by the oldest to the youngest member of the family. I have a little trick about lettuces that I would pass on to you so that you can have your greens living and full of vitamin C and chlorophyll and crisp and appetising: I do not pick a whole lettuce at all; I remove only the outside leaves from it, and eat these each day as I need them. When you remove the outer leaves, still leaving the lettuce growing in the soil, the chlorophyll is increased in the leaves remaining, which toughen up and begin to look like the outside leaves where most of the mineral and vitamin content can be acted upon by the light and the ultraviolet radiation from the sun. You can do this, too, with cabbages and brussels sprouts and heads of chicory, making an unusual salad of dark-green outer leaves chock-a-block with life, while still allowing the plant to grow on and repeat the performance.

The cucurbit family of vegetables—the pumpkins and squash and marrows and melons—will keep for some months once they are picked from the vine; but they are at their peak when eaten soon after harvesting: their taste is fresher, their flesh softer and more succulent and their vitality value to you greater. Fruit-trees take more of your time and attention if you wish to grow your own, and certainly cannot be grown and brought to fruiting maturity on a home-unit balcony—unless they are miniature cumquats. And what's wrong with a miniature cumquat? If you've never eaten a fresh ripe cumquat cut in tiny segments and tossed in with a few lettuce leaves and walnuts and cashews and a light soy-mayonnaise dressing, then it's high time you did. And you could try a lemon-tree in a tub. Feed it well and love it dearly and you'll be surprised how many golden lemons it will give you. You can't very well have a pumpkin vine trailing from your balcony down to street level if you live nine floors up, but you can grow decorative pots of Tom Thumb tomatoes at either side of your front door, and the harvesting you can do from these will supply you with piquant and eye-pleasing salads. Toss a few of these tiny brilliant ruby-red tomatoes with little melon balls, or with steamed new potatoes, throw in a sprig or two of chopped fresh parsley and perhaps a few dill seeds from your spice jar, and dress it lightly with a soy mayonnaise or a light lemon and oil mixture.

Salad vegetables come high on our list, because they grow so fast and mature so quickly with much life-energy. You can eat them for every meal if you wish; you can add them to any other dish you make; you can eat them after only a minimum of preparation and with no cooking, and they will please both the eye and the palate, a most necessary combination to set the salivary glands to work producing enzymes to deal with digestion.

Fruits and vegetables are lumped together here as good food, and I have chosen only a few to discuss more fully, to distinguish facts from fads and truths from half-truths.

TOMATOES

Some people believe tomatoes are good for rheumatism or arthritis; others are convinced that they have the worst possible effect. So I'll give you facts and let you make your own decision as to whether tomatoes are for you or not.

Although tomatoes have a pH reading of 4.24, which is about the level of a medium-acid fruit, they are alkaline in their body reaction and decrease the acid level. Tomatoes have all the minerals except sodium, high quantities of them in a fairly correct balance. They are well supplied with sulphur, silicon and bromine, and there is a trace of cobalt. Sulphur is the 'broom' of the body, sweeping out and cleaning up the débris; silicon is a mineral that can help to correct a calcium metabolism gone awry, as we find in both rheumatism and arthritis; bromine is a glandular system regulator and a stabiliser of emotional patterns and to some extent of hormone levels; and the trace of cobalt acts to destroy random cells wherever they occur. There are small amounts of vitamins A, B and C in tomatoes, and the digestion period is about two hours. They are low in calories and therefore low in energy value, so they are not what you could call an energy food. But they do contain about half the quantity of protein that is in potatoes, so they have some claim to being a balanced food.

The acids concerned are citric, mallic and oxalic, and the 'don't-eat-them' people claim that the high acid content cannot but worsen the arthritic picture. As W. S. Gilbert wrote so truly, 'Things are seldom what they seem', and the acids in the tomato even add to its usefulness in combating the deterioration that takes place when arthritis and rheumatism have become chronic. Some of the discomfort experienced by arthritis sufferers after eating tomatoes can be attributed to the 'stirring' going on in the stiff and crippled joints as the silicon gets to work trying to undo and loosen. There are two distinct forms of treatment for chronic arthritis: one is to halt and if possible undo the damage done, and this can be painful; the other is to stabilise the degeneration and give pain and discomfort relievers—without, however, gaining any improvement. If you want to undo arthritic damage and regain mobility in stiff crippled joints, you must be prepared to experience all sorts of elimination processes that may sometimes be really uncomfortable.

Gardening books give contradictory advice on growing tomatoes: some say you must feed them heartily, others tell you never to touch them. I have experimented by growing several isolated pots or plots of them, and treating each pot or garden bed differently; and to my amazement I've found each plant produces the same amount of fruit with roughly the same amount of growth. So I am convinced that the health and vigour of a tomato plant is in the seed stock from which it came.

There is said to be a greater vitamin C content in tomatoes when they are staked high and presented to the sunshine when ripening time is near; and it stands to reason that the more the sun's rays can penetrate the better the quality of the fruit. Allow the tomatoes to ripen on the vine rather than pick them green and let them ripen on the window-sill where they tend to ripen in patches. Pick them when they are a clear vermilion red and eat them within five minutes if you can. The difference in flavour speaks for itself.

LETTUCE

Lettuce is slightly acid in itself, but its body reaction is neutral. It takes over two hours to digest lettuce thoroughly. It has no fats and very little protein or carbohydrate, and it contributes bulk and all the benefits of green leafy vegetables, such as folic acid, calcium, and iron. Unlike some other green vegetables it is remarkably rich in silicon, and worth eating as a regular salad vegetable for this reason alone. It should be eaten by arthritic and rheumatic suffererers so that its silicon can gradually stabilise or improve their calcium metabolism. The combination of chlorine and sulphur in lettuce (together with its high water content) cleanses and purifies, sweeping waste matter quickly and efficiently through the system and out via the kidneys. Lettuce also contains bromine in such a form as to be a mild sedative, and some people find it pleasant to chew a few lettuce leaves or brew a cup of lettuce tea before going to bed. Make this tea as you would any herb tea: put a good handful of fresh, crisp lettuce leaves into the pot, pour in boiling water, let it stand for five minutes, and strain out your lettuce. Or just chew a few leaves instead.

POTATOES

It may be because potatoes are relatively cheap, or because everyone is used to them, that they seem an unexciting vegetable, apt to be ignored in terms of their benefits to health. A potato with the skin on, cooked in a vegetable-basket steamer over a little water, sprinkled with vegetable salt and perhaps a film of butter, or sprinkled with parsley or chives or a dusting of kelp granules, can be the most important part of a vegetable meal. Potatoes are particularly rich in potassium, with benefit to kidney function, and also in sulphur, that cleansing agent. These minerals occur mainly just below the skin, So that peeling before cooking means you are throwing them away. There are traces of vitamins A, B and C in potatoes, and the B and C are reduced even further when they are cooked in water. But we are not seeking vitamins so much as minerals.

Potatoes have not such a high water content as most vegetables, and the main thing against them in most people's minds seems to be their carbohydrate content. But we owe the potato an apology: its carbohydrate is only in the medium range; there is more in parsnips, more in kelp, more in all the dried beans and all the grain products, and very much more in nuts. If you are a weight-watcher you can do yourself more harm by eating a handful of nuts than by eating a whole baked or steamed potato. In our Western pattern of eating, lack of potatoes in the diet can produce a mineral deficiency. They are one of the best sources of minerals we can eat.

Apart from what we should or should not eat, there are few of us who don't enjoy potatoes. They give us a warming, comforting, home-by-the-fireside, dinner's-on type of feeling, and there are so many ways of cooking them: from the *Salz-kartoffeln* of Germany to the pan-fried potatoes of the Mediterranean, from the baked potatoes of England to the steamed, herbed potatoes of France or the buried-underground-in-hot-stone-ovens sweet potatoes of South America and the Pacific Islands. Their reaction in the body is neither acid nor alkaline but neatly neutral; they are lower in protein than many vegetables and can be included in commonsense amounts in low-protein diets. Their digestion time is approximately two hours. Those who cannot stand fats in the diet can leave off the nob of butter and eat them steamed rather than baked, confident that they are low in fats and will not upset the liver.

The sweet potato is one of the most valuable vegetables, yet it is not often included in our diet. The tuber must not be dug until it is fully ripe, otherwise when it is cut ready to cook it oxidises frantically and its food value deteriorates, as well as its taste and appearance. Growers should be made fully aware of this. The sweet potato is high in calories— those units of heat and energy—but it still has only about one-fifth the calorie- or energy-value of nuts.

The sweet potato does contain oxalic acid, but it also contains all the minerals and all the vitamins—every single one of them. It is exceedingly rich in vitamin A, which is one of the hardest-to-get vitamins in our usual food, and since the water content of sweet potato is low its vitamins and minerals are concentrated so that we don't need to eat very much of it to get a goodly quota. It has a fairly slow digestion time, and it takes about three and quarter hours for its benefits to be absorbed—so that when the more quickly digested foodstuffs are absorbed and gone the sweet potato is just beginning, spreading our nutrition over a longer period. Its reaction in the body is neutral (it does not tip our acid/alkaline balance at all) and it is one of those delightfully versatile vegetables that can be used with either sweet or savoury dishes. My grandmother had a sweet-potato pie recipe I have unfortunately lost, but I remember it contained pumpkin and melon skins and spices and seasonings. You can eat sweet potato cut in chunks and baked in a vegetable oil, or you can steam it and add sauces, or dice it and frizzle it quickly over high heat in olive oil, or deal with it any way your fancy or your recipe-book dictates; but I would *not* advise you to eat it raw.

The heat and the hunger satisfaction that potatoes give can stop you eating all those useless calorie foods containing refined sugars and starches. Your carbohydrate balance is thrown out by eating the wrong sort of carbohydrates. Any fighting Irishman will tell you that potatoes, like bread, are the staff of life; and when your diet is properly balanced otherwise, and compatible with your style of living, your energy requirements, and your individual metabolism, potatoes will not add one iota to your weight.

CITRUS FRUITS AND JUICES

If you are an orange-juice fan and go for it at the first sign of a cough or cold, you no doubt believe that its virtue lies in its high vitamin C content. But have you ever realised that the virtue of the juice cannot be compared with that of the whole lemon or orange or grapefruit?

Lemon juice is extremely low in calcium content: the lemon fruit with the peel and all is nine times higher in its calcium level. If you are eating citrus fruits to get the calcium you must work your way through the whole fruit or drink nine times the amount of juice. When you eat the lemon with the skin you are getting three times the iron, the same potassium, three times the sodium, double the vitamin B, nearly double the vitamin C and two and a half times more protein than if you just drink the juice. You are also getting some fat from the lemon oil, fat that is a useful fat. Lemon juice contains twice as much citric acid as does the lemon with the peel; the juice is a high acid that is processed to a slightly lower acid level in the body; but the lemon with the peel gives an alkaline reaction, most helpful if you have a cold which produces loads of acid mucus in your body. The whole lemon is far better for you than the part of it you get in the juice. Excess pure citrus can tend to corrode teeth that are not as strong as they ought to be, because of a diet of bland foods and processed mixtures that don't need chewing.

Citrus fruits all contain citric acid that can be damaging if the juices are consumed over a long period in concentrated forms without stepping up calcium levels or repairing damaged teeth. To preserve or restore health to the teeth you should chew a whole citrus, or at least a lightly peeled citrus. (It's not easy to eat your way through all of a sour lemon each day.) You can save the peel and shred it finely, or grate it beforehand, to add to stewed fruit, fruit salads, sauces, curries, or any other dish that is improved by the zingy flavour.

The same applies to oranges. The content of vitamin C and other vitamins is the same whether you eat a peeled orange or drink the juice; but the mineral content is quite different. You get twice the iron, more phosphorus, four times the calcium, more protein, and a slightly higher energy level in a peeled orange than you do in the orange juice. From a highly acid pH value of 3.9 a peeled orange changes in your digestion to a slightly alkaline pH of 7.1; orange juice changes from a pH of 3.76 to a pH of 4.5, which is still a very acid reaction. So eating a lemon, or having lemon juice with the pulp and peel added in a glass each morning, can be beneficial for arthritics; but the juice of oranges is a different story. Far better to eat the peeled orange if you have any high-acid condition of disease.

There is less vitamin C in grapefruit than there is in lemons, the same amount of vitamin B, and the fruit goes from an acid pH value of 3.5 to an almost neutral pH of 6.4 as it digests in the body, irrespective of whether you have the juice or the whole fruit. You get twice as much iron and twice as much calcium if you cut the grapefruit into wedges and eat it with a little bit of the white pith attached; but all the other minerals are the same, and grapefruit could be called a 'perhaps' fruit if you have high-acid disease conditions.

Citrus fruits are invaluable when your nose, throat and sinuses are choked and painful and full of mucus, for all citrus fruits have astringent properties: they tighten and contract mucous linings to enable you to breathe more easily, they loosen the mucus from the membranes so that it drains more quickly and the 'dog's disease' is banished in a shorter time. The high vitamin C content of citrus fruits certainly helps the elimination processes in colds and flu; but you would need to eat a case or more of oranges each day to get the massive amounts of vitamin C required to correspond with an injection of the vitamin or a 'high C' type food supplement. On the other hand, your body is better tuned to react to natural vitamins and better able to absorb the entire amount of them; so you can still drink your lemon juice (from now on knowing you should make it with the shredded lemon peel added) and feel you are doing something to chase your cold out of your body.

APPLES

If you eat apples with their skins on you will be healthier than if you peel them and throw the peel on the compost heap. If you peel them you lose some of the magnesium, sulphur, silicon and bromine that is close underneath the skin—these

vital minor elements in the major element metabolism—
and you halve the vitamin A content and lose a great deal of
the vitamin C. Apples differ from citrus fruits in that you
get almost as much of everything in the juice as you get in
the whole apple—with the exception of magnesium, which
drops by half when the apple pulp is extracted to make apple
juice. But an apple a day, while keeping the doctor elsewhere,
has one characteristic that is important to people in a high
acid state; after it is processed by the stomach its pH value
goes from 3.55 to 2.22, an increase in its acid content. This
may deter you from eating too many apples if you are arthritic; but for those of us who are not there is great virtue in
the apple reaching the intestines in an acid condition, for
intestinal flora cannot perform efficiently unless they are in
an acid medium. Don't mix up your stomach and your
intestines: the stomach is an entirely different section of the
body, doing entirely different things. The intestines, both
large and small, are parts of the bowel, and are completely
separated from the stomach biochemically, functionally and
anatomically. 'Pains in the stomach' often really mean 'pains
in the upper part of the small intestine'. We are talking here
about bowel flora, which need natural acid conditions to
function correctly. This is why apples are so beneficial for
people who have chronic constipation: they are a means of
reactivating the bowel and replacing harmful bowel flora with
a better class of bacteria altogether, so that natural bowel
movements can be restored.

Apples also give us what we lack so much—something to
chew. The chewing reflex and the hunger reflex are closely
linked, and sufficient chewing can suppress hunger; sufficient
hunger-satisfaction can suppress the need to chew. If we fill
ourselves with heavy, starchy processed foods to satisfy the
hunger reflex we have little need for chewing, and as we chew
less and less the chewing reflex becomes to a certain degree
atrophied so that we find we cannot chew raw foods if we want
to. On the other hand, if we make a practice of eating foods

in a fresh, raw state, as unprocessed and unsoftened and unblended and unemulsified as possible, our chewing instinct is strongly developed and our hunger reflex easier to satisfy.

GARLIC

While every German fräulein is evaluated as a cook on the individuality and perfection of her apple strudel, every Mediterranean cook is gauged by her skill in the use of garlic. You either like garlic or dislike it intensely, and its very pungency suggests qualities that cannot be ignored. You could call garlic the vegetable antibiotic: every bodily ill that can be treated by medical practitioners with antibiotics can have garlic prescribed by a naturopath or herbalist. The quantity of garlic needed varies, depending on the severity of the disease condition, and you can use it preventively, taking a small amount of garlic in your food; you can also use it in a heavy corrective dose of up to twenty garlic-oil capsules a day for infective diseases of a more serious kind. I have watched garlic bring down the temperature and boost the elimination processes of severely ill patients; it has stopped a flu-virus invasion in mid-battle; I have seen it remove considerable quantities of infective residues from a patient via the bowels and the skin and the kidneys and the lungs, clearing these vital organs for successful combat against the remaining infective agents; and, taking a few garlic-oil capsules every day, I feel it protecting me against the invading 'baddies' that surround me in my practice.

You can eat garlic or take the garlic oil medicinally in capsule form for any disease condition that could have 'itis' tacked on the end—tonsillitis, cystitis, sinusitis, bronchitis, vaginitis, gastritis, colitis, and many, many others. It acts as a cleanser, sweeping out the body with its high natural sulphur content (about 80 per cent of garlic oil is pure natural sulphur) and its iron and its calcium and other disease-fighting components such as pectin and enzymes. You might call garlic the vegetable guardian of human health: it not only combats and removes infective material, but also contains many substances that eat away chemically at cholesterol deposits.

To ward off many disease conditions at their onset, you can just eat a clove of garlic—and I do mean only a clove, not the entire garlic corm. Although this can give you a burning sensation on the membranes of mouth, throat and oesophagus, no actual burning takes place, and you can overcome the discomfort by drinking plenty of water with the garlic clove as you chew it. One patient of mine, a chef with a long-standing infective bowel condition, is in the habit of swallowing a clove of garlic whole whenever he can at his work, so that it arrives in his stomach relatively undigested and does not worry him and those around him with its odour. It also means that the garlic is readiest to go to work when it hits the area where it is most needed—his small and large intestines. While I would not recommend this to anyone with a delicate stomach, it is one way to overcome the odour problem. Another way is to buy from your health store a small bottle of aniseed oil, and with your finger place just a couple of crops on the back of your tongue. The strong flavour of aniseed will neutralise most of the garlic odour. A fresh clove of garlic is roughly equivalent to about four capsules of garlic oil in its effect.

This herb is used by naturopathic veterinarians as a worm preventative for farmyard animals and household pets. You can keep the animals healthy with garlic chopped up in their daily foodstuffs, and they seem to relish it, especially if they are off colour.

The only people who should not take garlic medicinally—or in any form—are those with degenerative or diseased conditions of the liver, gall-bladder, bile duct or pancreas. One action garlic has in the body is to stir the bile flow, and all this churning about of bile fluids can make such a person feel nauseated if he has eaten garlic. If this is happening to you, it may be wise to have your liver and gall and bile systems checked thoroughly so that any early damage may be repaired and correct function restored, after which you should have little trouble eating garlic if you wish.

You can grow garlic yourself. Buy a full, well-rounded corm from your greengrocer, peel off the outer row of cloves, and plant them about 25 centimetres apart. You should be able to harvest mature corms from these after twelve months; but if you leave some of them in the soil for a second year, or even longer, the size and health and pungency of the corms will be much greater. Garlic also conditions the soil in which it is growing, because of its antibiotic and antiparasitic qualities. Plants set out from the outside row of two- and three-year corms can produce a tremendously powerful batch of garlic.

There are so many foodstuffs in which garlic can be used as an added flavour that it seems a shame not to use it whenever possible. If you start with just a slight flavouring in soups and stews and rice dishes and salads, your family will not feel suddenly assaulted by the strong flavour.

Some companies insist that their executives have a blood cholesterol check each year to ensure that they are fit and able to continue a responsible job; and taking garlic could be one way of keeping the bloodstream free from the excess of this substance that either wrong processing or over-consumption of animal fats can cause. Such business men should frequent restaurants for their business lunches that lean heavily on garlic in their specialities; and eat it at home too, together with other members of the onion family. Boiled onions would have saved many heart attacks in the group of people most prone to them—those overweight, physically under-active, overfed, overdrunk and oversmoked individuals who clog up altogether in a heart-disease picture. The plain old-fashioned boiled onion every couple of days with a meal can help tremendously.

Although it is better in general to eat fresh garlic, it is necessary to consume quite a quantity of this to obtain sufficient garlic oil for therapeutic rather than preventive treatment. You can buy garlic-oil capsules from your health store —the more concentrated form is easier to handle. I prefer to take the capsules regularly, because otherwise I'd not get round to eating enough garlic each day; and I prefer to leave some of my plants in the garden to do work in the soil for me underground. You would need to have your entire garden planted all over with garlic corms to have sufficient to take medicinally.

The only infections that do not respond to garlic are those of a fungous nature, such as tinea and ringworm and the infections under the fingernail sometimes called whitlows.

Some people complain that garlic gives them diarrhoea; whereas garlic can be used as a herbal treatment to condition the bowels and reduce diarrhoea. What they are experiencing is not an infective type of bowel disease but a purifying, eliminating getting-rid-of-rubbish process that is removing the accumulated wrong sort of débris left over from wrong health habits. Some people also complain that if they take garlic for bronchitis it makes them cough even more. They are right—it most certainly does, and they have to cough and keep on coughing until all the phlegm and yellow or greenish mucous débris is removed. As my grandmother used to remark when any of the family did become ill, 'It'll be worse before it's better'—and she was right. There's no point in saying, 'There, there', and giving them a nice bland cough mixture that will anaesthetise the throat and bronchial area and still leave the entire respiratory system full of infection, inflammation and pus. Which would you rather have: a short period of discomfort while the rubbish is removed, or a longer spell, much longer in many cases, with a disease that can progress to chronic disability? Garlic is a mighty stirrer: it goes in there fighting, and it doesn't stop churning round until the job is done and there is no further need for it, except in a much smaller dose to stop the next bug hitting you.

I do not know what bacteria and potential disease conditions garlic has removed from my body; I only know they are not there now. How stupidly blind it would be to say, 'I won't take advantage of all garlic's blessings, because it doesn't smell nice.'

SEEDS

Almost every seed, particularly the seeds from grains, can be sprouted to provide a tiny edible vegetable. This sprouting process is the simple act of galvanising into life the compact little reservoir of life substance found in every seed. Most of you have eaten bean sprouts, the pale Chinese delicacy that goes with chicken chow mein and many other Oriental dishes, and there is nothing to stop us copying this piece of Oriental good sense. Amongst the commonest grains and seeds there are those that will sprout and be entirely and delectably edible. In the dormant seed there are no life processes, and it takes water to free into solution the tiny powerhouse of chemical combinations in the seed. Now, as the sprout shoots, it begins to manufacture vitamin C, and when the first two seed-leaves have grown there is a maximum quantity of this vitamin present, completely alive, wholly pure, utterly digestible, ready to be absorbed. When these two little leaves sprout from the pale, thin stem and the seed below, chlorophyll has arrived in the plant by the action of light and moisture, and this chlorophyll is at its most concentrated peak.

One of my favourite seeds to sprout is that of the fenugreek plant, the seed that gives the strong curry flavour to curry powders and pastes and that promotes perspiration and therefore the cooling of the body and the removal of waste products through the skin. The seeds send up their sturdy sprouts, as do most seeds, in a matter of three to four days. If you have ever sprouted seeds you will have had failures owing either to lack of regular washing of the sprouts as they grow, or to leaving them a little too long before eating, until the seed begins to rot, having done its job of giving life to the new sprouting plant.

Sprouts must be eaten within twenty-four hours of that pair of seed-leaves appearing green and full of goodness at the tip. Don't buy a bagful of the little mung beans (the green form of a variety of soy bean) and tip the lot into a baking-dish or some big tray-like vessel: you will either be giving away bags and bags of bean sprouts to all your friends and neighbours, who must then eat them within twenty-four hours, or you'll leave them too long and they'll rot. If you buy your seeds from a good supplier or a health store where you know that the goods are fresh and freshly bought, then you can be sure of at least 80 per cent germination from the seeds and grains you sprout. Less than 50 per cent germination can often mean that the original seeds have been standing in somebody's warehouse or on a shelf for over twelve months.

Keep sprouting seeds out of direct sunlight; but most seeds will sprout better in warmer weather or in a warm corner in your kitchen, since warmth speeds up the molecular activity within the cells. It is possible to sprout seeds all the year round. The colder temperatures in winter mean that you have a slightly longer time when the sprouts are at their peak, and their germination period can be four to five days.

Most of the grains are easy to sprout, and the easiest of the lot is wheatgrass. Freshly sprouted wheatgrass is one of the finest sources of both vitamin C and chlorophyll—that substance present in small amounts in all green growing things but in considerably larger amounts in the newly sprouted seeds.

The seeds germinate so rapidly that you will feel you have to plant them and stand back to watch. The shoots seem to turn green and grasslike within a matter of hours. I have one container, marketed by a Swiss firm, with layers of plastic circular shelves that fit one on top of the other: and if I make the mistake of putting those wheatgrass sprouts anywhere except on the top shelf, they lift the other shelves up as they grow vigorously and sharply green within three days.

Wheatgrass is blessed with a vitamin E content that can do apparent miracles in your digestive system, as well as in the garden and on the anti-pollution front. With all the minerals, the vitamin E, and the other balanced vitamins that it contains, it is one of the most compact, cheap, available, and natural sources of goodness. You can even add chopped wheatgrass, the green, growing tips of the wheat scissored off with care as they grow, to your drinking water, be it from a fluoridated water supply or no. Under chemical analysis you would find that with magical and astonishing ease the water no longer contains any trace of free fluorides, these having been converted into harmless compounds by the wheatgrass tips. I know of people who take little packets of fresh wheatgrass with them when travelling, even when going overseas by air, and they dump a little pile of wheatgrass into every liquid they are given on their journey. They even take jars in which to sprout seeds and put them on their bedside tables in hotels, so that a fresh supply of this prodigal helper is always available.

You can sprout mustard and cress, you can sprout millet and lentils, and most of the dried beans, including soy beans —and what a complete food a soy-bean sprout is! You can sometimes get fennel seeds to sprout, and aniseed seeds. If you are lucky enough to have a herb garden you can experiment with many of the seeds, and you will find that the edible ones add all sorts of piquant flavours to a green salad.

Another of my favourites amongst the sprouters is alfalfa ('alfalfa' if you follow the American custom; lucerne if you are British; but exactly the same stuff), for together with its splendid sprouting qualities it has another important use in the diet—it is highly alkaline. Most sprouts are alkaline at their peak and begin to turn acid as they age. Alfalfa sprouts could well be on everybody's menu in these days of increasing arthritic and rheumatic conditions, which we inflict on ourselves with our indulgence in white sugars and starches, leading to acid tissues and the beginnings of an arthritic pattern. It's simple enough to eat a few alfalfa sprouts from the container as you trek to and fro across your kitchen floor, and it's even simpler to drop a handful into the salad bowl each day and know that your family is dealing effectively with possible excess uric acid.

As far as I know, it is only in our civilised, enlightened Western world that people eat things they know to be bad for them. We have the knowledge and the choice; we know there are foods we need to provide an environment in which, both chemically and anatomically, we may continue in good health. Why do so many of us persist in refusing to provide for ourselves the foods we ought to have? A father provides for his family in many ways; but, in spite of her access to knowledge, how rarely does his wife give her family the best possible opportunities for good health! You can say, 'It's hard to change one's way of thinking, it's hard to get the family to eat "rabbit's food", and harder still to make them believe it's good for them.' Anything worth getting takes time and effort; and once you have used natural foods, natural sources of energy and fuel, you will find your family beginning to look like a family, not a collection of caged animals. And your time in the kitchen will be halved.

A sprout is a perfect form of balanced food. All the minerals are there in their purest form, and when light has begun the photosynthesis cycle and put chlorophyll there as well this ensures that the entire substance of the sprout will be absorbed and assimilated by the body. You are getting the vegetable side of seeds; and you are still getting, on that third or fourth day, the entire protein content of the seed as well. A soy-bean sprout contains a balance that could not have been worked out in any but a Divine laboratory to maintain abundant health.

Growing these sprouts is simple. You can use any of the

sprouting trays available through your health stores, or a wide-mouthed jar (preferably of glass; it's chemically inert) or a glass dish. You put seeds sparsely in the container, add enough water to wash them and swizzle them around, then drain off the water. The mouth of the container is covered with cheesecloth or coarse muslin—some material with a mesh open enough to let air and water through easily, but not to let the sprouts out. Each day you repeat the simple ritual several times: add enough water to wash the sprouts thoroughly, then up-end the jar and drain off the water. Enough fluid will be left adhering to the seeds and the walls of the container to begin and continue the sprouting process. This washing is essential: without it the sprouts will be checked in their growth or tend to go mouldy in the stale water still adhering to them from the day before. Two washings are usually sufficient each day.

SOY BEANS

Soy beans contain about one and a half times as much whole protein or complete protein as cheese; about twice as much protein as meat, fish and beans; and about eleven times as much as cow's milk. They contain not only the maximum proportion of amino-acids found in any member of the vegetable kingdom, but almost the exact balance of these amino-acids found in meat. I have often heard vegetable proteins described as incomplete proteins, meaning that they do not contain the complete balance of materials necessary for correct protein digestion; but this does not apply to soy beans, which could be called the 'meat that grows in the ground'. The carbohydrate content of soy beans is only about one-half of that found in other dried beans and grains; so they will not put weight on those who worry about weight from carbohydrates. They also contain only a little starch, so they can be eaten in diabetic diets and diets in which starch has to be eliminated or cut down. They are rich in calcium, phosphorus and iron in their dried form, and the oil from soy beans contains vitamins A and D, as well as E, F and K. The green beans that are picked in their live state, and not dried but either sprouted or steamed, contain vitamin C as well. Soy beans also contain lecithin, which acts as emulsifier of fats and controller of cholesterol metabolism. Being alkaline in their body reaction, having potassium in their alkaline salts, soy beans can be eaten by those suffering arthritic conditions, and can be used as a source of grain or flour material without adding starch and carbohydrates.

The hard little cream-coloured bullets of dried soy beans turn soft and edible after about forty-five minutes of pressure-cooking—my favourite way to do them. Whatever you do, soak the beans overnight or for several hours before cooking, and use the soaking water to cook them and, if possible, to serve with them. Much of the heavy mineral content from the beans is in the water. The flavour of this bean may prevent its being generally eaten in our pampered society where nothing seems palatable unless it tastes of sugar or salt. You have never really experienced the true pleasure of eating until your palate has gone back to a natural selection mechanism by which the taste of a lettuce grown on clay can be clearly distinguished from one grown on acid soils. We have lost that discriminatory sense of the flavour of good food. Soy beans on their own could turn a Westernised palate right off; so you don't serve them on their own at first, but with all sorts of natural flavours and seasonings, such as a little tomato and onion, fresh herbs and grated apple, soy sauce and a touch of basil, or a few sprigs of mint and a dash of lemon juice. One of my preferences is to mix the cooked beans with sultanas and basil and garlic, then the whole lot is quickly sizzled over a good heat in a spoonful of soy oil. Stir the beans briskly, or they will burn and become inedible. Just before serving mix chopped fresh tomatoes through the beans.

The Chinese delicacy called bean-curd, a soft, custardy, white, cheese-like substance, is made from soy milk, much as cottage cheese is made from cow's or goat's milk. Soy milk comes from boiling the soy beans in water until they soften completely, then straining and reserving the liquid. This is allowed to curdle and the curds are hung in clean muslin or cheesecloth to drain. The resultant slithery curd must be kept under water, in the fridge if possible, until you are ready to eat it—within twenty-four hours.

Soy flour can be added to any recipe that uses flour, in a proportion of about one part of soy flour to about four or five parts of whole-wheat flour, and there is no appreciable difference in taste. If you go through your natural foods cookbooks carefully you will find many recipes in which soy flour on its own is used, and the taste is delightful. The somewhat bitter taste of soy can blend with other flavours to provide sharpness and interest even in standard recipes. Soy flour has about fifteen times as much calcium, seven times as much phosphorus, and ten times as much iron, as ordinary white milled flour. Its overall mineral content is four to five times as rich, and its B-group vitamins about eight times higher than in the poor residues we have left to us in standard white flour. Soy flour holds and retains more moisture than white flour and therefore gives you a moister finished product. It is fluffy and a little lighter in weight, and it can perk up all sorts of standard family-favourite type dishes. Just as with any other new habit, it's a good idea to start gently: don't give the family soy pancakes for breakfast, soy muffins for morning tea, soy-bread sandwiches for lunch, soy biscuits for afternoon tea and soy crêpes for their evening dessert, all in one day! Take it slowly and try a little at first with their favourite dishes so that they can remark on the flavour; then add a soy dish to a particular favourite meal; and gradually you will find you can introduce soy beans to the menu with confidence. There are excellent cookbooks with many and varied soy-bean recipes.

No doubt you have all tasted soy sauce sprinkled over Chinese food; but have you tried wholemeal spaghetti bolognaise with a little soy sauce on top, and soy 'mincemeat' instead of steak? If you put a little basil through the 'meat' sauce with the tomato, and a dash of lemon juice with the soy sauce over the top, you have an exotic dish that is basically nutritional; and if you sprinkle pure grated parmesan cheese over the top of this concoction you are assuring your stomach of enough calcium to digest it all very happily.

It is sad that 'good' food is so often thought to be plain food or uninteresting food. There is no reason why meals should be dull just because we have halved the preparation time; and adding fresh herbs and vegetable flavours can do wonders to make a simple meal into an exotic adventure. You may think a sauce is something to make a 'dry' meal go down more easily; but there are sauces that are a whole meal in themselves or that add their own contribution to a basically good food. If you have pine nuts from your health store and fresh basil in a pot beside the kitchen door, with first-pressing olive oil from your speciality food store and a little lemon juice from the tree down the backyard, you can have a sauce to grace any rice or farinaceous dish that is not only nutritious but contains more goodies than the main bulk of the meal. Chop a few roasted hazelnuts through cashew butter and mix in with it a teaspoon of lemon juice and a few scrapings from a dried vanilla pod, then swirl all this through a little natural yoghurt with slices of fresh peaches, and you have a dessert that makes Peach Melba seem dull. If you chop a sprig or two of lemon thyme and dark green eau-de-cologne-mint leaves through it as well, you have an individual flavour hard to duplicate in any traditional way.

Many mothers interested in natural and nutritional foods are weaning their babies from breast milk not onto animal milk but onto soy milk. From all the reports I have had, it seems to be a thoroughly satisfactory substitute, and from the contented babies there have been no complaints. This type of weaning-food leaves little waste residue material, so motions are fewer, sometimes making a new mother fear that her child is constipated. This is not so: the soy is just completely absorbed, and the alkaline reaction tends to produce less nappy-rash, too.

KELP

Here is a natural good food if ever there was one—kelp, coming straight out of the sea and being dried as its only processing. The kelp we buy from our health store or vitamin supplier is usually from one particular species, *Fucus vesiculosis*. Its other common name is bladderwrack. This particular seaweed grows in many parts of the world, in a slightly different form perhaps but under the same botanical banner, and it is a logical food for obtaining in our diet some of the heavy minerals and trace elements that have been washed off our mountains and down our creeks and out to sea ever since the earth cooled. The human body still needs these minerals, and we still have access to them if we use seafoods, particularly from the deep-sea areas where all the heavy minerals finally finish up. There is iron at the bottom of the sea, and gold and silver and titanium and vanadium; there is nickel and silicon and zinc and boron; and these elements are found in minute traces in each human organism. It seems they were put there for some purpose that we in our ignorance have not yet discovered. We know iodine keeps our thyroid gland from developing goitre, but we do not know how our body uses silver or gold, or even if it wishes to have either of these elements or needs them at all. They are there anyway, and if we wish to give our bodies an environment in which they can function in health and vigour we should attempt to give them, through our food, fuel that corresponds to their internal climate.

This is one of the reasons I give to vegetarians who deplore my enjoyment of deep-sea fish as a weekly or twice-weekly meal. The enormous benefits of eating foods coming from the deeper regions of the sea quite nullify, in my mind, the odd worry about metal containers rusting away with their loads of industrial or radioactive wastes, or about parts of space-ships hurtled back to earth and fragmented into smashed molecules somewhere under the ocean. It's a mighty big ocean, still very much a natural, primitive area; and seaweed, or kelp, comprises most of its primitive vegetation. By eating kelp we may be nourishing ourselves not only with scientifically analysed and understood minerals and vitamins but with the heavy elements that enabled primitive forms of life, even human life, to change and mutate and acclimatise and eventually cover this planet.

Kelp has about the same amount of vitamin C weight for weight as do oranges. It is also high in vitamins of the B group, particularly B_{12}: there is almost as much B_{12} in kelp as there is in the liver of animals and from animal sources. There is vitamin E and vitamin K there too, and although science would have us believe that vitamin D does not exist as such in the vegetable world, there is evidence that it does. Kelp has proved to be a preventive and corrective agent to stop rickets in animals under research conditions, and the researchers have assumed that vitamin D must be present in this marine vegetable.

The iodine found in seaweed comprises compounds of iodine amino-acids—that is, the iodine is in the same form as that associated with the thyroid gland. The thyroid does not have to process it or change it; it goes straight into the stomach and the bloodstream, and homes in on the thyroid where it is available for use immediately. It follows that kelp is a good natural food supplement for those who live a long way from the sea and cannot get iodine in any other natural form, and for people who do not eat fish or shellfish and need the salty tang of the sea in their veins.

Kelp contains a form of vegetable sugar, but this sugar does not raise the blood sugar levels at all; so kelp is a good nutritional supplement from which diabetics can safely gain their mineral requirements. Some fat and some protein also exist in seaweed, but it is a vegetable protein and contains only one or two of the unsaturated fatty acids. One of the best qualities of kelp is its ability when growing to absorb all the minerals in the sea around it, sometimes in a concentration several thousand times higher than that of the sea-water itself. Seaweeds are primitive vegetable growths and have existed as such unchanged, having very little relation to our land plants. They do not produce flowers or seeds, and they grow without root nourishment, attached by 'holdfasts' to rocks and the sea-floor. Every part of the plant can manufacture its own food. Someone who takes kelp in his diet for the first time may not notice any benefit for some weeks, even a month or more. It seems that kelp in the intestinal tract creates its own climate in which a particular type of bacterium of the friendly variety then multiplies. As soon as the bacterial count is high enough, then for ever afterwards every grain of dried kelp you eat will be completely absorbed. Here is an example of how an environmental change can occur internally to adapt itself to a particular external condition. The body is such a marvellous and infinitely complex organism that it can even alter its functions within limits, so that a new foodstuff or a new set of living circumstances can be dealt with and adapted to.

Kelp grows at an enormous rate. It can be harvested by a particularly simple method, that of hauling up to the surface from small boats long trails of slimy kelp and slicing off a metre or two, then allowing the plant to slither back again into its deep-water bed. This top-growth of the plant, being closer to the ultraviolet of the sun and containing more life and nutriment, is much more valuable medicinally than the lower part of the plant nearer to the ocean floor; and about three days later the metre or so that is hacked off will have regrown. When you think of the countless miles of ocean forests of kelp that can keep producing a complete food for mankind at this rate, you wonder why we are pumping artificial fertilisers into our weakened soils in an endeavour to feed ourselves.

I often prescribe kelp for patients with stubborn, vague symptoms that resist other forms of natural treatment. Such patients react favourably to kelp, and I suspect that one of those trace minerals somewhere in its composition is responsible, providing a trigger of some sort or a missing element that sets the whole works off in perpetual motion once more. Seaweed can be added to the diet of most domestic animals, and my little Corgi dog really relishes her meat when a light sprinkling of kelp granules is added. Dairy and beef cattle react very favourably to kelp, with a general improvement in condition and an increase in fertility and health of the young. The milk output in dairy cattle can be increased by using kelp as a supplement, particularly when the animals live a long way from the salt air. You may wonder why grazing animals need salt sometimes and are given salt licks to keep them healthy. I hope they are given a salt lick made from sea salt, which comes coarse and pure and unrefined straight from the sea with nothing added to it and nothing subtracted from it. What is keeping our cattle healthy could be those trace minerals found in kelp that are also found in lesser concentration in sea salt. Our cattle may no longer need salt licks or salt supplements if they have kelp in their diet in sufficient quantities.

Australian kelp can be particularly fine in quality, and that gathered commercially from the South Coast of New South Wales is amongst the world's finest. Traditionally, Norwegian kelp is the most expensive and the most highly prized in the Western world, but our South Coast variety I have found particularly potent and remarkably flavourful; and I can get it fresh and properly processed. The only thing that is done, or should be done, to kelp when it is harvested from the sea

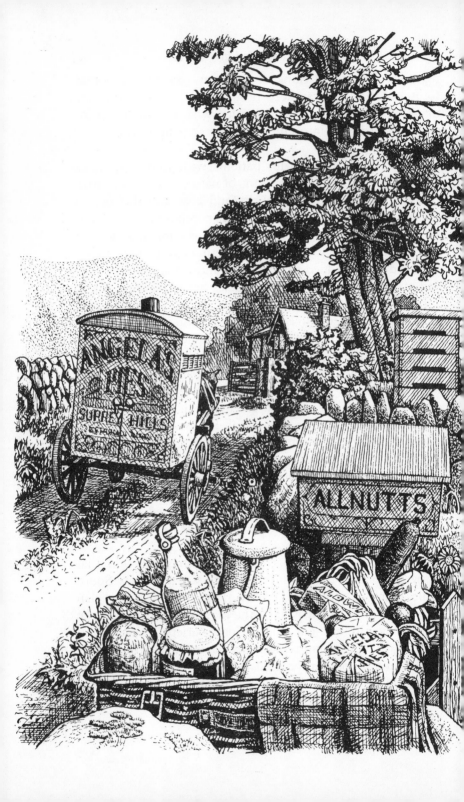

is to chop it up and dry it. It is not washed, and should not be washed (if you harvest some from the beach after a storm and dry it yourself). You will find no impurities in the dried material, no pollutants, for kelp seems to have an effective barrier in its cells to anything that is not natural. We have here the perfect vegetable, but because it is hidden from us underneath the waves we have not used it—unlike our more economically minded neighbours who live closer to Nature and draw their living from the sea.

I was given a small packet of Japanese sea lettuce by one of my students, and it has kept in a screwtop jar for over three years. The flavour is just as fresh as the day I first opened the packet: and since most of its value is in its mineral content it is still just as good now as it was when I took the first mouthful. I use it thinly sprinkled over rice dishes—particularly if they have a seafood base such as fish or prawns or Tasmanian scallops or mussels—and the somewhat oily oyster flavour blends very well.

BANANAS

If you enjoy eating bananas and you are putting on weight it's not the bananas that are to blame. Though the banana is an appetite-satisfying, filling food, it has a low calorie count, only about 85 to 90 calories for an average-size banana. This means that it is lower in calories than a good-size serving of cottage cheese, and it is also lower in calories than many of the so-called low-calorie foods that often replace it. These calories are not empty ones like those in white sugar and white starch products; they are full, nutritious calories, and the carbohydrate from bananas when they are ripe is not only readily digestible but helps the body to store protein.

If you eat bananas (say, one or two a day according to size) you are getting about one-fifth of the daily amount of vitamin C that the mythical 'average' human being should have; so you can eat bananas to supplement or even replace citrus fruits if you do not like these or should not have them. There is a good proportion of the B vitamins in bananas, too, particularly B_6 which they have in comparable amounts to liver meats, the best source of B_6. Then there is vitamin A in very large quantities; so you can eat this fruit if you are allergy-prone: indeed, it is often used naturopathically as a dietary method of controlling allergic-type reactions. There are three essential amino-acids in bananas as well.

Bananas do not contain any of the so-called 'bad' items of diet. Their fat content is minimal and is mostly unsaturated. They contain only a minute trace of sodium, and are highly suitable for people on a low-salt diet; and those with a gall-bladder or kidney or heart condition may still eat bananas and enjoy their unique flavour without worrying. There is absolutely no cholesterol in bananas. There is calcium and phosphorus and iron—even more iron than there is in an apple—and under the skin of unripe bananas is to be found an antibiotic-type substance, which may account for the Pacific Island custom of baking green bananas in their skins and eating them this way. Like apples, bananas contain pectin, that wonderful digestive enzyme substance that aids in digesting any other foods eaten at the same time, and they are most useful in normalising bowel function for patients with either chronic constipation or chronic diarrhoea. On a diet of bananas together with other food, the acidolphus bacteria in the intestine rise in number; and since these are among the 'good' bacteria intestinally, bananas go part of the way that sour milk products go in providing a better climate in this vital part of the body. For sufferers from colitis and stomach or bowel ulcers, bananas are valuable because of their non-irritant qualities and their ease of digestion.

You can suffer allergy symptoms if your body will not tolerate one or other of the amino-acid groups found in animal protein, and here we find bananas most useful: their protein content is of a benign nature, and allergy sufferers find that adding bananas to their diet helps to reduce the distressing symptoms of running nose and puffy eyes and the sniffling miseries these disease symptoms can cause.

Diabetics can eat bananas safely, for the blood sugar levels are thereby neither raised nor lowered. They have also been found useful as an item of diet for those unfortunate children suffering from coeliac disease, an allergy to wheat products.

There is some basis for the misinformation on the subject of bananas that leads one to suppose they could be fattening. It is true that a baby introduced to bananas as one of its first foods at weaning time will rapidly gain weight. But such babies have usually been badly fed, or the mother's health has not been good while she has been breast-feeding, and her nervous or emotional state has made the child tense and underweight. After weaning, this type of child can rapidly gain in weight and improve in temperament if a banana, mashed on its own or with other foods, is included in its diet each day.

People who retain fluid because of kidneys that are under-functioning or sluggish or slowed by residual disease symptoms can benefit greatly by eating bananas, and in this case a banana diet can contribute to loss of weight.

So if you had no bananas today, it might be a good idea to have some tomorrow!

DAIRY FOODS

Milk

Cows, like most other things, are not what they used to be. The dairy cows we see paraded around our agricultural shows have very little in common with the earlier models of their species. First of all they are much larger and heavier; secondly, the size of their udders is enormously increased; and thirdly their life-span is about 20 per cent shorter than it was only thirty years ago. Are we going forwards or backwards? Maybe the cow our grandmothers used to milk produced a higher-grade product than what we get from the dairies today. You can't increase milk production from the same size herd seventy-five times without having some doubt about the quality of the milk produced in such volume. I remember drinking fresh milk an hour or two after it had left the cow, and although I was only a child of seven or eight at the time my taste buds tell me I have never since drunk anything that could be called 'real' milk. That cow may have given only a fraction in volume compared to present-day standards, but the concentration of milk solids and vitamins and minerals—the *quality*—was so much better.

Contact with the viruses and bacilli and bacteria that man has a nasty habit of gathering to himself caused many and varied diseases in the bovine world; and Science has had to come to the rescue with antibiotics for everything from mastitis to tuberculosis. So milk cannot be what it used to be. For one thing, there may be so much penicillin and antibiotic-type residue in the milk from the dairies that cheese refuses to result when cheese should result. Not only have the 'bad' bacteria been eliminated but so have the good ones, and the various strains of yeasts and moulds and fungi that give cheeses individual and characteristic flavours just can't grow in their antibiotic environment. So cheese manufacturers have to resort to artificial methods of maturing cheese and the product, though acceptable in flavour, is nutritionally debased.

We are constantly exhorted to drink more milk. But why should we, and what does it contain, and what has happened to it before we bring in our morning milk-bottles? Did you know, for instance, that milk contains hormones, a fact about which little is known except in the nutritional field, but about which more should be learnt before we label it as good for everyone from weaned infants to great-grandmothers? The milk comes from the cow's teats and falls into sterile containers. What agents have been used to sterilise those containers? There is bound to be some residue left on the container walls of a powerful disinfectant or germicide which may or may not be harmless to humans. The milk is then loaded into bulk containers that have also been hosed out with disinfectants and germicides and in which milk from many different dairies and hundreds of different cows is mixed before it reaches the bottling or packaging plant. If just one cow in one of those herds has symptoms of disease that contaminate her milk the whole of the sloshing white load will be contaminated before it reaches the depot. With so many new and resistant viruses and bacteria about, who is to say whether the contents are still sterile? The dairy farmer, the tanker operators, the processing plant personnel, our friendly milkman: we have to depend on them all, and I am certainly not criticising their cleanliness or conscientiousness; only pointing out the many things that happen to milk after it leaves the cows' udders. When a calf suckles milk directly from its mother the milk enters the calf's mouth uncontaminated and sterile, and this is the only way it can be sterile. If it is exposed to the air, even for a short time, bacteria and other deteriorative agents can invade. Milk is, as you know, perishable stuff—a prime growing medium for fungi and bacteria and the less exposure it has to the air the better. It is better kept covered at all times, and decanted only as you need it.

Milk is pasteurised at the bottling plant, which means it is heated to kill the bacilli and bacteria present; but there is always a tiny residue of bacterial matter that survives this heat. This happens by the very nature of bacteria, which are cussed little beasts refusing to conform to all the rules humans lay down for them. If the milk comes to you in clear glass bottles, you will by now know that its vitamin content is altered and lessened by the sunshine and light filtering through the glass before you store the bottles in your fridge.

Whole milk, just as it comes from the cow, contains the fatty acids and vitamins A, E, D and K; so there is obviously much to be said for drinking it as long as you can be sure that its benefits outweigh its drawbacks. Milk contains high proportions of calcium—which all of us need and most of us lack—and it is worth considering as a source of this mineral. But you must be aware that the calcium in milk can precipitate in a manner distressing to a human body that is not in a fit state of health to process it correctly. Calcium precipitation, upsetting the metabolism, can be responsible for many ill-health conditions from gallstones to arthritis. But there is a way out for people with this disability who insist on drinking milk: a dilution factor. Calcium precipitation should not occur if you remember to drink at least two glasses of water for each glass of milk. This separates the molecules somewhat and dilutes the quantity and therefore the absorption rate, so that your body can handle the calcium metabolism more efficiently.

Milk is said to be a necessity in our diet for several reasons, reasons we should examine closely for their soundness. The most important is the maintaining of the vitamin B level necessary for the complete health of the nervous system. Vitamin B can be manufactured in the intestines when lactose is present. Lactose is the name given to the sugar of milk, the energy part of it, and you might say, 'Well, if I drink enough milk my intestines will be healthy and will produce a lot of vitamin B.' This unfortunately is not so unless the bacteria in your bowel are benign and healthy enough to enable the process to take place. If you are eating the wrong foods, such as white bread and white sugar and the heavy starches and carbohydrates, if most of your food is of the processed, pre-packaged, manufactured variety, your bowel will be supplied with bacteria of a very different sort, most of which will be harmful or potentially harmful and have no effect whatsoever on the lactose from the milk. However, if you drink or eat sour milk products lactic acid is produced from the lactose and a better type of intestinal bacteria is achieved.

If you are a very active person and you enjoy sport or

physically demanding, energetic occupations such as gardening, walking, jogging, swimming or board-riding—or if you happen to be a milkman running briskly for many hours between his customers and his van—you will produce lactic acid in your muscles. Problems can arise when there is too much lactic acid in the muscle fibres, where it is produced anyway as an end product of the breakdown of glycogen, the muscles' primary fuel substance. If you are a physically active type of person your muscles can clog up from an overabundance of lactic acid. You will have to run twice as fast, or mow a bigger and wilder patch of lawn at twice the rate, to burn up this excess lactic acid, or your muscles will gradually become fatigued to the point of becoming flabby. This may sound the exact opposite to what you have always been told about milk being a body-builder; but I am giving you the facts and sifting the evidence to show you what is going on in our bodies after we drink a glass of milk. If you like to separate your own milk to make your own cottage cheese and drink your own whey (the clear liquid remaining after the curds have risen to the top), 70 per cent of the lactose of the milk will be in the whey; and since whey has been spoken of as a nutritious food this may appear to be a contradiction. Whey contains not only high calcium and lactose, but also the correct proportionate amount of sodium, and by the time it has reached the stage of becoming whey it has absorbed from the air or from other sources sufficient bacteria to render it slightly sour. These are in the main beneficial bacteria, and the souring process changes the biochemical picture from a hard-to-digest cumulative one into a relatively easy-to-digest, constructive one.

Some of the claims made for milk are quite true and provable, one of them being that it makes young bodies grow at a faster rate. It was noticed when comparisons were made that infants weaned from mother's milk onto cow's milk grew much faster than those weaned onto other products. Since cow's milk is intended for calves, which grow and gain weight four times as fast as human children, this is not surprising. But it is not necessarily the biggest and bouncingest baby who is the healthiest, and health is what we are concerned with, not the breeding of a bigger and supposedly therefore better race. Only 30 per cent of milk drunk is digested within one hour from the time of swallowing it, whereas some 90 per cent of the soured milk products like yoghurt and buttermilk and whey (bacterially pre-digested) are processed by your stomach within the first hour. You get no chewing with milk, or with any other fluid you drink either; so the advocates of a 'milk lunch' are only doing part of their nutritional home-work when they say that it completely satisfies and provides you with all you need for the rest of the day. You must satisfy your chewing instinct sufficiently or your body does not feel it has eaten enough in quantity; and drinking a glass of milk —even milk enriched with yeast or wheatgerm or whatever else you care to throw in it like honey or protein supplements in powder form—will not give you complete hunger satis-faction by any means.

There is a place for milk as well for any other food as long as we know what that place is, and what its value is to us. The soured products made from milk are of enormous worth to us, and to have soured milk we must perforce start from fresh milk.

Devotees of skim milk say that if you drink this milk with a great proportion of the butterfat removed you can do yourself no harm. But exactly what nutritional value are you getting in that milk? As soon as you remove the fat globules from whole milk you remove most of the fat-soluble vitamins as well—vitamins A, E, D and K. Vitamin K is the one you need to prevent clotting-type diseases such as strokes; vitamins A, E and D are valuable to all of us and we cannot do without them. Does the skim milk give you any goodness at all? Only if you must be on a fat-free diet. But then you are better off going without milk altogether and making up your fat-soluble vitamins from vegetable oil or natural sup-

plement sources. Nature designed milk as she did, and man's
meddling does not seem to me to produce a better product.
Once you take away a part of a whole food, any part, you are
losing that vital balance.

I drink the occasional glass of milk and find it relaxes me
when I come in from the garden slightly hungry and slightly
thirsty, with my muscles beginning to ache. (You will understand now why a glass of milk at such times can be of nutritional value.) However, I usually prefer my milk soured to
some degree and in some manner so that my body will not
have to work nearly as hard to process and absorb it. If I
want to go out in the garden again to work after a short rest,
I shall not have a glass of milk. It is only at the end of my
working spell that I can afford to have my muscles relax and
grow tired. The warm glass of milk at bedtime can do the
same thing for some people.

Buttermilk

Buttermilk is a low-fat product, the residue of milk after the
butterfat has been removed in butter production. If you have
ever drunk a glass of buttermilk fresh from the churn, as I
have in a small Swiss village, you have tasted one of Nature's
delights that has many nutritional virtues. It is another
soured milk product, and it is generally made commercially
from pasteurised or skim milk so that you know immediately
what vitamins you are *not* getting. But because buttermilk is
soured you know also that your bowel is going to benefit,
and your digestion, from the increased calcium absorption
in your stomach and intestines. Our buttermilk is from commercial sources and I have no idea what processing steps it
has gone through; but it is still one of the better type of milk
products, and the less preservative it has with it the better.

Whey

Whey is the clear liquid left when the milk curdles naturally
and the curds rise to the top of the container ready for you

to make your own cottage cheese. Whey can be made in any household by the simple method of letting milk stand without refrigeration. Bacteria from the air and any bacterial agents present in the milk originally will sour it, and the clear liquid left under the curds is about 70 per cent lactose, together with much of the milk protein and the greater part of the minerals, plus water. Whey has been used therapeutically for everything from the complexion to ingrowing toenails, and health benefits are claimed for it in many diseases in which basic nutritional deficiencies occur, or when nutritional imbalances have helped to establish the disease. It has been found that while an infant is nourished on mother's milk, there is only a simple bacillus, *Bacillus bifidus*, in the intestines as bowel flora. This is a similar bacillus to the *Lacto-bacillus bulgaricus* present in various sour milk products such as buttermilk and yoghurt. As soon as the child starts to eat other foods, particularly those highly processed products out of jars and cans that our culture insists are baby food, the bowel and intestinal flora change rapidly and the beginning of the long self-poisoning that is civilisation's nutritional lot is under way. Even in an adult, too much animal protein can build up harmful strains of bowel bacteria, as can too much carbohydrate material. The bowel flora can grow and multiply beneficially and produce all that necessary vitamin B only when it is given fresh fruits and vegetables and soured milk products proportionately to other foods to maintain the ecological balance in that part of our anatomy.

Yoghurt

Yoghurt is one of the most ancient processed foods known. From the time man began to domesticate animals he has used the milk of the animals to drink. It is more than likely that the greater part of the milk consumed was some form of soured milk, the milk that had gone slightly 'bad' when there was no ice or refrigeration. Every country and every culture has its own type of soured milk products, but many of these are lumped under the one heading and called yoghurt. You can make yoghurt from the milk of any animal: it has been made from cow's milk, buffalo's milk, sheep's milk, goat's milk and even, in the southern part of Russia, from mare's milk. Milk was drunk freshly taken from the animals, and that left over was stored in skins and leather bottles for later; and, as you can imagine, it went 'off'. Thus was discovered a nutritional wonder—the multitude of good bacteria and bacilli that could help man process his food and make it more easily digestible and palatable by using Nature's way and not his own. You can even make yoghurt from camel's milk if you have a camel in your backyard. This may be of value if you can't stand fats in your diet, since camel's milk contains no butterfat whatsoever.

The principal fermenting agents in 'bad' milk are *Lactobacillus bulgaricus* and *Streptococcus thermophilis*. These are both 'good' bacteria in spite of their fearsome names, and yoghurt has a nutritional value so far in advance of the original milk whence it came that you may never bother to drink a glass of milk again. All you need to make your own yoghurt is one container of store-bought yoghurt, some fresh milk and constant low heat. There are good books available from your health store that tell you how, and you can buy constant-heat machines that make the process easy and mistake-proof.

Many people tell me they can't eat yoghurt because of its acidity, and there is always a reason why a body refuses a certain food: in this case it happens because the bowel is so rotten with putrefaction and the stomach so lacking in calcium, so tense and tight and irritated, that the goodness of yoghurt is just too much for the system. The body rejects this dramatic change of environment, this complete reversal of bacterial population, as something so new and different as to be revolutionary. Bodies can get used to frightful nutritional inadequacies if they persist long enough, and even a good change can be initially upsetting. This is why I never advocate any extreme diet changes like prolonged fasting, or sudden switches from eating four chops every day to complete vegetarianism, from eating Western-type sausages-and-veg. meals to eating Eastern-type brown rice and curry spices. The body would be quite justified in rejecting such a sudden and complete change of fuel. Do things slowly and gradually over a longer period of time, and the body will take much better to whatever is the new fuel. A bowel over-loaded with toxic putrefying matter and bacteria of the wrong sort is going to have to work very hard and do a lot of eliminating once the good bacteria and the right sort of foodstuffs hit it; so it is going to be a change accompanied by some discomfort or even by acute discomfort until the new pattern settles down.

You are all acquainted with the fruit flavours added to commercial yoghurt, and sometimes the different acids of the fruit so added react adversely in storage with the lactic acid unless proper care is taken in the manufacture: this is where you get 'blown' yoghurt cartons. You can get over this problem by buying plain yoghurt without any added flavours, and adding your fruit and your honey and a touch of lemon juice immediately before eating it. There is no such thing technically as a plain 'bad' yoghurt. It will go on getting more and more sour the longer you keep it and will eventually become quite unpalatable.

Yoghurt is milk plus. There is up to 35 per cent more protein in yoghurt than there is in the milk from which it came, and it still contains the calcium, phosphorus, vitamin A, thiamine, riboflavin and niacin. As soon as you eat yoghurt rather than drink milk you double your absorption of calcium, and you put live bacilli and bacteria into your bowel to create a healthy environment in which the constipation or diar-rhoea, the colitis or gastritis a putrid bowel can breed should not occur. Yoghurt neutralises excess hydrochloric acid in the stomach, so it can be very beneficial for sufferers from stomach ulcers, increasing the calcium absorption to help in the healing of the ulcers while neutralising the acid irritation that can give so much pain and discomfort. Yoghurt can also lower the blood alcohol level after you have been imbibing, so you may like to mix up a new drink like yoghurt and cherry brandy and a dash of lemon, or whisky à yoghurt with ice. You can use yoghurt, too, as a morning-after remedy if you have wined and dined a little too freely.

Yoghurt can even be used as a vaginal douche, its good bacteria counteracting the many and increasing infections prevalent amongst our free-living younger folk: everything from monilia and trichomonas to the nasty new herpes-type infection that is plaguing both males and females. A yoghurt wash can soothe the sore, irritated vaginal lining, and its good bacteria can fight against the invading troops of the more damaging variety.

Yoghurt made from goat's milk is more easily digestible than that made from cow's milk, for the fat globules are of a different variety and size and break down into absorbable portions more quickly and easily. You can wean a young baby straight from breast milk onto soured milk products and ensure that the bowel of the child and the intestinal flora remain in the healthy state that mother's milk maintained, without the deterioration often found in a baby's condition at weaning time.

Butter

In so-called civilised countries about half the milk produced from dairy herds goes into the making of butter. Butter is one of the products for which I fail to see the initial need. It used to be thought of as a food for the 'poor' people, and in medieval times it was eaten only by the servants and the peasants while their lords and masters dined on oil-prepared and high-protein foods. You can eat it or you can leave it alone according to your beliefs, but its main function still seems to be to make a slice of bread go down more easily.

Some say that butter is bad for you, others assert that

butter is better for you than its substitutes. You must decide yourself which you prefer—or if you wish to eat neither. It may come as a surprising thought, but there is really no need to butter your bread, if you are still a bread-eater. If the bread has a taste of its own, it is indeed preferable not to butter it, just putting some sort of filling on top of it and another slice to make it into a sandwich. The habit of buttering bread must have happened when our taste buds and our digestive processes started to deteriorate as we got lazier and lazier and more civilised. A piece of dry bread became the all-time low status-symbol.

Most of our present-day butter is made from soured cream; but it is still possible to buy sweet butter made from sweet whole cream, and the difference in taste is very obvious. In commercial butter preparation, salt is added to prevent moulds and other deteriorative processes, and sodium carbonate or calcium carbonate is added to neutralise the salt. The butter may have 'bleaching' processes carried out on it somewhere during its manufacture, and may then have colouring added to it to make it look like butter again. It is possibly the most mucked-about-with simple food, and the one that we can most do without in our diet.

It's true that you do get vitamin A from butter—that is, the actual vitamin itself as well as the carotene for your body to make it from. It is also true that the vitamin A content varies, depending on whether it is butter from cows fed on summer or winter pasture, on rich pasture or on poor. Indeed, the vitamin A content of butter is a nutritional barometer showing the quality and strength of the dairy herds. You also get vitamin E from butter, and vitamins C and P; and vitamin D itself, the sunshine vitamin, is present, as well as traces of the B group and quite a bit of iron. All this, of course, applies to pure butter, and not necessarily to the butter we buy commercially prepared. It is so obvious that the quality of the end product depends upon the health and vitality of the animal producing it that you would think this would be the first point made in the promotion of dairy foods. But there is no mention of what herds the butter has come from, what agricultural conditions those herds live amongst, what type of season the area has had, and what type of feed supplement was given to those animals.

It is better to use unsalted butter, if you must use it at all, in your cooking, or if you still like buttered bread. If no salt is added there is no need to add substances to neutralise the salt, so that's two additives that are not present: and the most part of unsalted butter marketed is packed in some light-repellent material that tends to reduce any rancidity occurring from bad storage or from overheating.

I shall not join the argument as to whether margarine and other butter substitutes are better than butter for sufferers from high blood-cholesterol levels. High-cholesterol sufferers can do all sorts of things by varying their diet, but their levels of cholesterol can be reduced only by correcting the original causes, most of which are not related to their dairy-food intake.

A telling survey was conducted some years ago by the School of Public Health at Harvard and the School of Medicine at Trinity College in Dublin. This study used Irish male twins, and in each case one of each pair had stayed in Ireland and one had migrated to America as an adult. The nutritional and health states of each twin were compared to find what nutritional facts or factors of any kind were now present even though the twins had been reared in Ireland under identical conditions as boys during their basic growing periods. It was found that the Americanised halves were generally more overweight, had a higher and earlier incidence of heart disease, had higher blood-cholesterol levels, a much higher level of disease, particularly chronic disease states, and were in general far more unhappy and very much more unhealthy than their Irish counterparts. The dietary patterns of both sides were studied and it was found that the Irish half of each pair lived on all the so-called wrong foods—

large amounts of potato, home-made bread and dripping, milk and butter and cheese and eggs, and high carbohydrate intake in the way of porridge and cereals—yet were happier and healthier than their Americanised brothers. The nutritionists concerned were forced to agree that diet *on its own* had no influence whatever on the health or disease conditions of those tested, but that other factors were involved too; the most different of these being in the realm of exercise. Although the Irishmen at home in Dublin or in other parts of Ireland were absorbing all the so-called wrong foods in large quantities, they were living simpler lives, most of them on farms or in farming districts where they walked a great deal and the air was fresh and clear, they depended entirely on their own efforts for their own rewards, and the overlay of civilisation was not so confining. The survey team conceded that this basic difference in exercise patterns and styles of living could be the major factor in the different health situations of each twin brother.

You can draw your own conclusions from this survey, but it would appear obvious that if you wish to eat a lot of this type of food, dairy products and carbohydrates, then you must change your way of living to burn up the excess energy and fuel in healthy outdoor exercise and simpler ways of living. The American half of each pair of twins was zealous in his consumption of low-cholesterol foods, butter substitutes, low-fat products and high protein staples, but mostly his wife drove him to the station in the morning, he sat at a desk, and spent the evenings gazing at television with a glass of something alcoholic in his hand.

I take no sides at all on the vexed question of whether dairy products can be classed overall as good or bad or indifferent foods. They suit some people and they do not suit others, and you will soon know they don't suit you if you become overweight and sluggish and lethargic and build up all manner of illness patterns that may not have occurred without this type of foodstuff in your diet. However, if you are a country man or woman who works hard out in the open sunshine and fresh air, if you use a lot of physical energy each day and you live simply and contentedly on produce from your own farm and milk from your own cows and potatoes from your own vegetable garden and eggs from your own fowls, then butter and other dairy products should not be harmful to you.

Cheese

I do enjoy cheese when I'm sitting with my friends around my table or in front of my fireplace talking at the week's end and relaxing in a cosy living-room; and this is the only time that my stomach ever says 'cheese' to me. Maybe it knows that the next day I'll be out in my garden working hard with a mattock or a hoe, mulching and digging and pruning and harvesting the bounty that my garden provides for me, and that I'll be working off that cheese I ate the previous evening.

Our present-day cheese is a far cry in most cases from its ancestor, the simple curded milk that was coagulated by adding rennet (a substance found in a calf's stomach) to the milk and then heating the whole thickened fluid to make hard cheese and to separate the curds and whey. I regard cheese almost as a separate section, and only vaguely as a dairy food, because so many things are done to it to remove it from the dairy-food family in the way of flavourings and moulds and fungus and bacilli injected into it to produce those multivarious flavours available from the cheese counter. The modern approach to cheese is to process it; and in most countries products thus made must be so labelled—telling you that what is inside the cellophaned, silver-foiled, chemically protected package is *something*, but not necessarily pure cheese.

There are as many different ways of making cheese as there are cheese varieties, and it has always been a simple article of diet for simple folk in simple cultures, the natural process of curdling and heating being explored, using a natural curdling agent from one of Nature's animals, the calf. We are using in this substance Nature's way of digesting milk for a calf, not for a human; so cheese is not necessarily easily digestible for us. But its flavour and aroma and sheer appetite-provoking tastiness make us want to include it here and there as an article of food. By the time it is artificially coloured, has had acidifying agents added to it, and emulsifying agents and hydrocarbons, perhaps in the form of colouring or flavouring or an artificial 'smoked' flavour... by the time it has been sprayed with a coating of wax that may have chemical additives in it to prevent other moulds and bacteria growing, by the time the entire container or package is again sprayed with a form of insecticide to protect it from vermin in storage...you can see that the product you are eating has again been got at in many different ways before it has reached your table, and cannot always be called cheese.

One of the best cheeses, if you are going to eat cheese at all, is parmesan cheese: because of its method of preparation and its natural long-keeping qualities, its dry, powdery texture and its hard, resistant and impervious skin, it is one of the safest ways of eating a cheese product without getting too much of a chemical feast in the process. Parmesan cheese is extremely high in calcium content, and this calcium is fairly easily digested for a cheese. It can be sprinkled on all types of dishes in its grated powdery form and stored for long periods without deterioration. You can extol the virtues of good old-fashioned English Cheddar, or Stilton in its stone jar; you can enjoy the subtler flavourings of Roquefort and Gruyère; or you may prefer the more natural cheeses, such as cottage cheese, which is only the curded part of the curds and whey, left hanging in a muslin bag dripping into a bowl for some hours to remove the last bit of watery content. Cream cheese is made not from the whole milk but from the cream or cream-and-milk, so it has a higher butterfat content and a smoother texture. Your guide in buying cheese should be, 'How was it processed?' How many steps did it have to go through artificially before it got to your table? Or is it of the variety where natural ripening and natural maturing has been allowed to take place—in which case it is almost certainly far more expensive but also of far more nutritional value?

Bread and cheese was the peasant's midday diet in most civilisations for centuries, and with it went a flagon of home-made wine. Cheese is rich in protein, undoubtedly, and in a concentrated form of protein as well, so you don't need to eat a great deal of it for your protein requirements. It is a whole protein from an animal source and is something you must consider to be a good food, depending as always on the amount eaten, and in what circumstances. If you are a seden-tary middle-aged accountant or a plump contented house-wife who prefers to sit and chat over a cup of coffee for relaxation rather than play a good game of tennis once a week, then you must relate your cheese intake to your life style. This goes for all the dairy foods: the more active you are the more you can handle them. If you have the type of daily routine where the only walking you do is from the front door of your home to your car, and the only off-duty relaxation you have is sitting in front of the television, you must think hard about how much dairy food you can eat and still remain healthy. An active, vigorous outdoor existence is what you need to burn off in a natural manner any excess waste these dairy foods can produce.

It sounds silly to say it, but if you are healthy you don't get sick; and if your body is healthy it can handle a reasonable amount of dairy foods. But if your body tends to produce excess acid residues (in such illnesses as arthritis, and in digestive complaints, liver weaknesses, sluggishness of the kidneys and the associated eliminatory channels) then the soft mucous linings of its openings and passageways will be constantly irritated; and when they get hit with a large wallop of dairy food they produce more mucus, and at an increased rate, to combat the irritation. The 'mucusless diet' routines you find in natural health publications suggest ways out of this; but my way out is to improve your body health first, and then adjust your dairy-food intake to your style of living. A healthy sinus or healthy bronchial tubes can handle a reasonable amount of milk or cheese without complaint; but as soon as that initial imbalance occurs, for no matter what reason, dairy foods are the first articles of diet to go under the axe.

When you think of mucus this way, as the first line of defence of a body that is out of balance, you will see that a good way to restore that balance is to cut out temporarily foods known to have the effect of increasing mucus production. When your body's equilibrium is back again and you are healthy enough to handle anything, you can go back to those foods again.

Dairy foods are as good as the health of the herds they came from and the care taken in any processing methods they undergo later. If you can obtain them in the purest available forms, without too much adding to and subtracting from, then you have a good simple staple food to be used in moderation and with knowledge of what effects it can produce in your body and of what nutritional value it can provide for you.

MEAT OR FISH OR BOTH OR NEITHER

Meat and fish are the chief source of protein in Western civilisations. Protein is the building material of the body, for new cells are made of protein and the body cannot be built without it. But a diet consisting only of protein foods would make you very ill indeed: for the body it is building must have cementing substances and structural reinforcing to hold it together.

So what about vegetarians? While I am not one, I do prefer a diet that provides protein very much more from fruits and vegetables than from animal sources. I may eat steak perhaps once a week, but am more likely to have brains or liver or kidneys; and I enjoy fish of all sorts and believe firmly that deep-sea fish is something without which a vegetarian cannot *easily* be healthy. Fish is not only a protein food but a valuable vitamin food as well, and the minerals it contains are essential. If you are not in a good state of health or your stomach is ulcerated, tense and irritated, you may find that meat protein gives your digestion a heavier job to do than other forms of protein.

The argument of those who love their red meat and eat a good-size portion of it every day seems to be that the protein in meat is a whole or complete protein. It is not the proteins as such but the components of these proteins—the amino-acids freed in the process of digestion—that circulate through the cells and do the real work. If you know which vegetables give you the highest protein count (or amino-acid count) you can include these in a vegetarian diet or eat them instead of meat protein every so often to provide a balance of elements for the digestion, ensuring that amino-acids are available. About eight amino-acids have been found essential for life and are present in meat in different quantities, depending on the cut. There are about another fifteen amino-acids that the body can make itself; but it appears certain that the first eight must be obtained from foodstuffs.

The amount of protein needed varies from person to person, and what may be insufficient for one person can be ten times too much for the next. The basic need for everyone is to have sufficient protein to replace the body cells as fast as they are being destroyed, supplying more cells so that the life-growth cycle is maintained. If the body is in a state of natural health, full of vitality and contentment, it is likely that less cell destruction is going on, and the need for replacement materials correspondingly less. But in every one of us, no matter how healthy, the processes of decay, destruction and excretion are going on all the time and cells must be rebuilt to maintain life.

In children and adolescents patterns of growth must be maintained and developed with particular care, to ensure that they progress healthily to maturity and become well-grown adult humans. It is for these young people that protein food can and must be used in the diet to maintain the balance of growth.

I have many vegetarian friends who are full of life and vitality; but I have equally many vegetarian patients who come along looking sickly and pale and lethargic. People who are vegetarians usually have a moral objection to eating any form of animal life, and some are even total vegans—eating no animal product whatsoever, no eggs, honey, milk or cheese. Such people must have adequate knowledge of what fruits and vegetables and grains and seeds and nuts contain, so that they can balance their meals to give adequate nutrition. Vegetarians who fail to remain healthy fail through lack of knowledge rather than through vegetarianism. For instance, soy beans are a complete protein, exactly the same as beef, and a completely nutritious food. And if you are a vegetarian who does not include soy beans in your diet you can well be undernourished.

If you have moral scruples about slaying animals to feed people, there are many valid arguments to convince unbelievers, and one of these is that many animals are killed when they are in a state of terror. Fear makes adrenalin rush out into the bloodstream and the muscular tension and corresponding biochemical pattern result in the animal's being in a thoroughly unnatural, unhealthy state when it is killed. The animal that walks down Death Row at the abattoirs to be hit on the head either by a captive bolt or by a sledgehammer, or whatever the humanitarian impulses of the killing-shed management provides, cannot be said to be in a good state of health. Animals that are hunted before they are killed, or that are trapped or snared, are in the same state—abject fear toughens up their muscles.

You may argue that this is all a lot of tommy-rot, and

that it would take weeks and months for an animal to become biochemically changed by fear and tension, but many of you know that the biochemical effect of panic and terror can be so instantaneous as to give immediate body reactions in animals, as in humans. If you then cook the killed meat in a variety of time-consuming or high-heat processes, it will be devitalised altogether, so that maybe that last piece of burnt charcoal-coloured steak from the barbecue is so extremely dead as to be utterly worthless as food. It is true that protein is not generally destroyed by cooking processes; not destroyed, no, but changed in a way that makes digestion of it slow and difficult. With all the other peculiar foodstuffs we put into our stomachs these days, anything that is going to make it a harder job to get nutrition into the body should be given a second thought before it is included too often in the diet.

It is not true that the more exercise you do the more protein you need. Those high-protein supplements carried by hikers and climbers and people doing endurance-type activity are not really as necessary to them then as they have been led to believe: while the endurance test is going on, they could be better off with energy-type foods such as carbohydrate products, and natural carbohydrate foods, than with concentrated protein foods. The protein would be more useful taken before and again *after* the trip, or climbing the mountain, or swimming twenty-eight miles, or running on the spot for four days—to repair and rebuild cells that broke down during all the effort.

Protein can also load up the excretory organs with heavy products not so easy to get rid of, and a vegetarian diet is certainly kinder to the kidneys and the bowels than is a high protein one. This is worth remembering if the excretory organs are choked or under-performing because of disease. Another fallacy is that by taking plenty of protein you can arrest the deterioration caused by age and progressively rebuild the body.

What has happened to the animals we eat before the chop or steak appears at the table? Beef animals and pork and veal livestock are artificially fattened on a force-fed, chemicalised diet much more now than they were twenty years or so ago. Chickens have hormone pellets embedded in their flesh to fatten them more quickly by artificial castration. Grazing animals are a little safer, but even they are given synthetic additives during the growth period; and the pastures have no doubt been crop-sprayed or dusted or fertilised with many and varied synthetic products in order to restore their depleted state. It is much easier for an animal to absorb synthetic harmful substances than it is for a plant, and animals and even insects absorb greater proportions of them than plants do. The plant will more often die, showing you quite obviously that it does not like these substances and cannot live with them accumulated in its roots and foliage, but the animal will absorb chemicals of a synthetic variety more readily and retain them in its flesh.

It is much better for you to eat organ meats—brains and kidneys and liver and tongue—than it is to eat muscle meats. The muscular flesh is more likely to be affected than the functional organs by what happens to the animal in the last days of its life. There are also more minerals and vitamins in the organ meats than in the steaks and chops and legs and shoulders. Organ meats contain a tremendous amount of phosphorus, as well as the iron found in most animal tissues. Meats also contain the B-group vitamins, and if you are eating no grain products at all you will find it hard to obtain sufficient vitamin B from dairy sources alone. Most meats are very high in this important vitamin, which vegetarians get by eating wheatgerm and yeast.

The liver and kidneys of grazing animals contain a good proportion of copper, the mineral we need in minute amounts for our iron and calcium metabolism. They also contain folic acid, the high iron and anti-abortion vitamin. Liver contains vitamin D and vitamin B and enormous amounts of vitamin A, as well as choline to regulate liver function. If you forgot all other meats and ate only liver and kidney, you would have a superb nutritional balance between your protein, your mineral and your vitamin needs. When I have been able to persuade my vegetarian patients who are looking seedy and unhealthy to take desiccated liver tablets they have never failed to correct the nutritional imbalance.

Meat of any sort has some calorie value, although it is low compared to that of carbohydrate foods; so you do get some energy and warmth from eating meat. The B_{12} vitamin so readily available in liver is something your family may be going without unless they are eating comfrey in enormous amounts to replace it. Liver is a complete protein and high vitamin food; but the liver being what it is—a magnificently complex and entirely self-contained biochemical factory—can be easily upset chemically by the hormones or antibiotics or artificial foods given to animals to increase their size and saleability. Chicken livers are splendid food, and if you can run those chickens around your backyard to grow naturally they can be killed for the table and their livers made into a paté that is nutritionally high-voltage stuff.

The leaner cuts of meat contain more protein than the fatty ones; and organ meats have scarcely any fat at all. They are also low in calorie value, so if you wish to lose weight, start off with organ meats as part of your reducing plan. Vegetarians are way ahead in their vitamin B absorption if they eat seeds and nuts and grain products; and if you have not been eating this type of food regularly no doubt your only sources of the B-group vitamins, so essential for the health of your nervous system, have been meats and some dairy products. Since vitamin B comprises a water-soluble group of vitamins, it should be obvious that boiling meats or steaming them will reduce the vitamin B content. Meats baked or grilled retain more vitamin B and the juices from the pan can be used for gravies. If you boil meat, be sure to add the liquid to soups or stews or sauces, for the vitamin B content, although much reduced, should not be thrown away.

Extremely high temperatures reduce protein value and content alarmingly; and it is also bad for meats to be pressure-cooked. Grill at a moderate heat and save the pan juices, and always eat your meat as soon as it has reached the point of edibility, not letting it become black and scorched and nutritionally worthless.

This does not apply to pork, because pigs, fed on slops and waste products, can be carriers of a parasitic worm that can deposit its eggs in human interiors; then the hatched worms can wind their way into human muscles, particularly those of the diaphragm. Eating half-cooked pork or salami sausage containing half-cooked pork may result in embryonic trichiniasis. The symptoms are sharp colicky pains around your diaphragm, diarrhoea and fever, loss of sleep and heavy sweating, and some muscular discomfort. These symptoms can also belong to many other disease states; but if you have been eating undercooked pork and they do occur, you should have a pathological test to see whether you do or do not have trichiniasis. If you do, and you wish to avoid the purging-type treatment given for this type of disease, just eat loads and loads of fresh garlic and take garlic-oil capsules over a long period of time—many months are usually required—to deter the *Trichinella spiralis* embryos altogether.

I believe that the publicity about mercury levels in fish has been grossly overplayed by the media and that fish is still one of the purest of all foods. Fish do not carry disease to humans; they do carry minerals and vitamins and protein and they carry them in a form that can be readily digested and quickly absorbed. This all applies only to *deep-sea* fish: if we come closer inshore, into estuaries and bays and harbours, we find a different kettle of fish altogether!

Fish from different parts of the world are surprisingly similar in their nutritional value, whether they are caught off the coasts of Japan or Norway or from the waters of the southern Pacific Ocean. The outstanding exceptions are cod and halibut, whose livers are packed solid with concentrated vitamins A and D. Ocean fish contain iodine in therapeutic quantities, just as kelp does, and fish, like kelp, is a good source of the iodine that many inland folk and isolated goitre-area communities so badly need. If you eat canned salmon, sardines, herrings and tuna, make sure you eat the soft bones as well. These fish, as well as giving you massive doses of vitamins, give you calcium and phosphorus in concentrated amounts.

Fish is low in calories, so you won't be adding weight, but will be getting some energy. I would always recommend fish as the first solid animal protein to be introduced into the food of an infant, with perhaps desiccated liver from animal sources as the second. It may be many months before muscle-meat protein can be added without overloading the developing digestion of the child.

Fish cooks quickly, and for this reason alone you could recommend it. If you live in Pacific Island areas, or in the Far East or Middle East, it is quite likely that the fish you eat will be raw or almost so, or perhaps soaked in some protein-digesting medium like coconut milk or lemon juice immediately after it is caught. Scandinavian soused herring and Japanese marinaded fish are excellent food, not being subjected to cooking processes at all. Fish contain calcium, large quantities of phosphorus, iron, and a trace of that all-too-scarce copper, besides a trace of magnesium and the iodine we have mentioned. Vitamin B is there in large amounts too.

Shellfish, with their magnificent flavour and taste, must now struggle for existence in polluted waters, being found closer inshore and therefore closer to civilisation's waste-disposal areas. It is still possible in some parts of the world to prise oysters from their shells on the spray-washed sea edges and eat them without any fear of contamination; but these places are getting fewer and farther between. Although water, if it keeps moving, can usually purify itself over a period of time, it is more and more likely that waters around our foreshores have not been given that time before another load of waste and pollutant material hits them. If you buy prawns or oysters or mussels from commercial sources it is more than likely that they come from fishing grounds not far from shore. However, I do believe that the shellfish are still, comparatively, more nutritionally safe than the flesh of land animals: the pollution they absorb from their feeding grounds cannot be so great as that deliberately pumped into land animals.

Pick your fish supplier with care—and if possible get your fish direct from trawlers, or from wholesalers or fish markets. Even fish can be got at by unscrupulous wholesalers and retailers: if they do not sell immediately they can be preserved for a little longer by using chemical sprays or adding chemicals to the tubs in which they are stored. Fish from a fish shop can be thawed out and re-frozen and thawed out and re-frozen before you buy it. But you must know the old safety principle with buying fish—look at the eyes: If the eyes are clear and full and rounded, you can be pretty well sure that the fish has been caught within the last twenty-four hours; if the eyes are dull and sunken away from the sockets, your fish could be very old and therefore very dead indeed.

To avoid deterioration of fish through transporting and selling and then retailing, it is sometimes frozen immediately at the wharf as soon as the trawler comes in. And if you want to buy fish as untampered with as possible, then frozen fish would probably be the next-best buy after fresh fish straight from the trawler. Fish with white flesh is usually more easily digestible; and the less oil the fish contains the whiter and more easily digestible is the flesh. Fish with a heavy oil content in the flesh, such as flounder and plaice and sole and mullet, have a more grey, leathery skin and a sharper and more pungent flavour.

It is seldom that you can buy whole fish with the entrails intact from your fish shop; but if you know your trawlermen well or catch your own fish, you can use the fish livers as the most nutritionally complete part of the entire creature. If you don't fancy eating them yourselves, give them as a succulent special treat to your dogs and cats, and don't forget that they like fish-heads too: my Welsh Corgi whirls about in extreme bliss when I come to her dangling a fish-head from one finger as her weekly treat. Down it goes, bones, eyes and all; and there's a very healthy little dog sitting here beside me now because she's nutritionally happy.

EGGS

There is still much to be learnt about eggs and the substances they contain, and about the role these substances play in human metabolism—as well as in the growth and development of the chicken that may spring from them if they are fertile. You could call the egg a seed, the germ of new life. We know that seed foods contain a vitality substance that can produce new, complete, whole entities of the animal and vegetable world; we know, too, that the good health or ill-health of the new entity is predetermined by the quality of the egg or seed. So the question here is not whether eggs are good food (they certainly *can* be) but whether their *quality* provides the nutrition we are aiming for.

You must bear in mind that the facts about eggs apply to eggs of top quality, to eggs from healthy fowls running about in the open air and sunshine, eating living insects and living seeds from living vegetation, having their diet supplemented by grain and green fodder from natural sources. Such hens almost always have (or had) a rooster with them. This natural balance produces a majority of eggs that are fertile, the hens being fertilised by the cock before the eggs are laid. And such eggs have the complete nutritional balance—the life and the structural framework for that life, the minerals and vitamins and proteins—and are worth their weight in almost any other good food you can name. But in the poultry farms of today thousands upon thousands of anxious, distressed, over-crowded hens have to be encouraged by perpetual light and calmed by soft music to lay their eggs, and the eggs are totally infertile. Whether such eggs can possibly have good nutritional qualities you must decide for yourself.

The life of the birds is considerably shorter when they are kept in batteries and artificially fed, and their eggs are a pale imitation of those with golden yolks and thick viscous whites from the backyard and farmyard poultry of yesterday. If you have ever eaten eggs from hens kept in such natural circumstances you will know how different they are and sense their quality as a nutritionally balanced, compact food.

Many people who love eggs for breakfast or any other meal have been told that they should not eat them because they contain cholesterol. I have already explained what cholesterol is, and how it is manufactured in the body, and which food-stuffs contain it. Certainly eggs do contain cholesterol; but they also contain lecithin in proportionate amounts, so that the cholesterol and its processing substance are together in the one food. This type of compact nutrition is simple, and you don't have to worry about what to eat with it or after it.

There is no vitamin C in eggs, but there is a good quantity of vitamin A and some vitamin D, and there are vitamins E and B, in particular biotin, which is in the egg white. There have been some popular-Press scares about how raw egg white or even cooked egg white can be damaging, especially for the kidneys, and as usual they have been based on misconceptions and half-understandings. Raw egg white, if you lived on a diet of nothing else but, would make you very ill indeed; but then so would a diet of nothing else but almonds or nothing else but figs, or nothing else but meat. There is a substance in raw egg white called avidin that destroys biotin, and it does seem strange that Nature should put a substance and its destroying factor both in the same section of the same food. This is one of the many things about eggs that are still not explained or understood. The egg contains all the essential amino-acids in the correct proportions, so that it is a balanced food in this regard; and one whole average-size egg would give you about 6 grams of protein—not enough to cover protein needs by any means, but contributing to them in a readily digestible form.

The shell of the egg contains calcium, magnesium and phosphorus, and if you have a kitchen blender you could very well crush and pulverise the shells of the eggs to provide an excellent source of these minerals. When the shell is crushed to a fine powder it is no different in consistency from any other fine powder, and can be added to flour and baking mixtures or can be mixed in small quantities with your muesli at breakfast time. The shells of any eggs you buy should be checked by you to see that they have a matte, dull finish. Any eggs that are shining and smooth have most probably been washed; and a dangerous property of the egg is that its outside covering is permeable. A certain amount of air penetrates the egg, and any liquid (some liquids more than others) can carry impurities with it through the eggshell. An egg is so susceptible a host for the growth of bacteria that many of our virus and bacterial agents are cultured in laboratory conditions by injecting them into eggs. Such a medium is very vulnerable. Even if you store eggs in the refrigerator—and it's best, if you can't gather them freshly from your own fowls—you should know that the eggshells will allow to pass through any odours or contaminating agents that are with them in the fridge. It is a pity that we usually have to keep eggs in this way, for every hour in storage decreases their freshness and life. Fresh eggs gathered from where the hen has laid them no more than a few hours earlier keep at the peak of their freshness for only about four or five days, and even each of these days produces deterioration in quality. One of the initial reasons for our commercial egg producers keeping hens segregated from the rooster (so that the eggs they laid would be infertile) was that unfertilised eggs keep much longer. The greater nutritional value of 'live' eggs has been understandably overlooked,

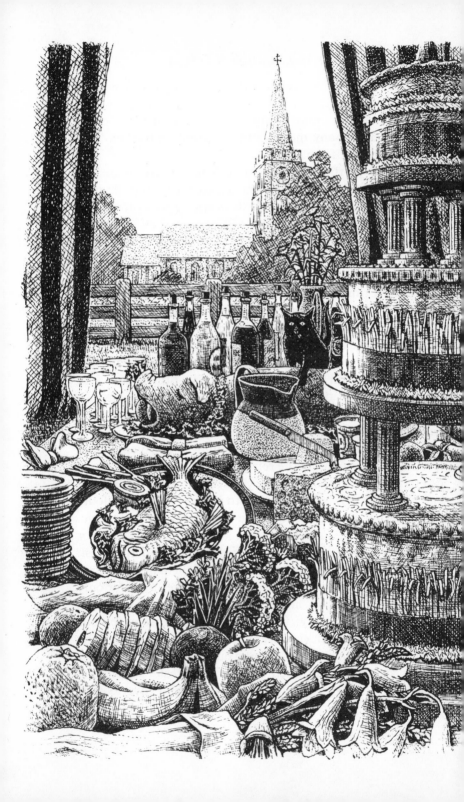

because the 'dead' eggs can be marketed in bulk and stored for long periods.

There is nothing to stop you eating raw eggs, as long as you remember that you eat both the yolk and the white together. Our diet does not naturally consist of a large proportion of eggs, in spite of their valuable properties. If you eat eggs for their high calcium content or for their protein, remember that there are substitutes to replace them entirely if you wish. For instance, eggs have the complete amino-acid count in the right proportion; but soy beans have twice the amount, also in correct proportion. The mineral content of eggs is exceedingly high, and most of them occur in the yolk, which is particularly rich in iron. The trace of copper so necessary for assimilating iron is also present, as are calcium and phosphorus and magnesium and chlorine, and a small trace of the substance that drives egg producers crazy—sulphur. Organic sulphur is the substance that gives egg yolk its colour, and that also, in Nature, begins to destroy the egg contents if they are not fertilised, or if the chicken is not developing correctly. You all know the smell of the hydrogen sulphide gas generated in a rotten egg!

Any eggs that are discoloured or blotchy should be discarded, particularly if the blotching is in the yolk of the egg. Specks of blood in the yolk do not necessarily mean that the egg has been fertilised and may result from the hen's ovaries being hormonally unbalanced by injections or pellets given to stimulate her to lay more. The white of the egg should be firm, not runny at all; and of course you know the old test for freshness: when the egg is placed in sufficient water just to cover it, it should not rise to the top. If it does, some hydrogen sulphide gas could be forming.

ANIMAL-PROTEIN SUBSTITUTES

Nuts

Nuts could be the answer if you wanted to live without a

refrigerator or a stove. Stored by Nature in thick shells, they are splendid food, and far better nutritionally when eaten stone-cold raw. The odour of roasting nuts in your department store may tempt you, but the cooking rapidly destroys their nutritional value. If you are going to eat nuts, eat them raw. Enclosed in their shells, nuts keep for many months, sometimes for years; and this means that you can buy them when they are cheapest and store them and have them all the year round if you wish. Once nuts are out of their protective shell, they will soon become gluggy and tasteless or verging on rancid in flavour; so shelled nuts must be put into airtight jars immediately and kept there until you are about to eat them. The constant handling and unpacking and repacking that goes on in stores and warehouses ruin shelled nuts; so it is better to buy and store them in the shell.

Different kinds of nuts contain different minerals, absorbed from the ground and from the air as the tree grows and fruits; and different portions of the same nuts may have a different vitamin and mineral balance covering a whole range of nutrients. There are a few damaging substances in some nut shells—the extremely high tannin in walnut shells, and the irritant materials in cashew-nut shells, for instance. We are almost never able to buy cashew nuts in the shell for this reason, the nuts being stripped before they are allowed to enter the country; so this nut will always have less than its full nutritional value when you buy it. Many nut crops are chemically freed from their shells before being marketed, so if you buy kernels you may unwillingly be buying a harmful substance rather than a healthful one. Some nuts are soaked in lime and others are freed by acid from their shells, exporters using whatever is the fastest and most economical method.

Nuts are not complete protein foods, as eggs are; and although they contain what is in effect the seed of the plant they have not the complete amino-acid count found in animal products. They are high in vegetable oils, those vital oils so necessary as an alternative to fats from animal products; they

are high in concentrated protein, but quite low in carbohydrate; and they can be a valuable substitute for sugars and
starches. You do not have to eat very many nuts, for their
contents are exceedingly concentrated.

There is a false belief that nuts are indigestible—and nuts
can be indigestible if they are not properly crushed and
masticated by the teeth before they enter the stomach. It all
goes back to our lazy chewing habits. Stomach acids are able
to handle nuts very well when they are broken down into
small portions; but they are not able to cope with or break
down nuts that have been insufficiently chewed.

Nuts do not contain uric acid, nor do their end-products
break down into uric acid, as those of meat can; so arthritics
can eat nuts in preference to meats and keep their tissue-acid
levels lower. All nuts—except perhaps peanuts and walnuts,
which give a slightly acid reaction in the metabolism—have
an alkaline residue. So people with tissue-acid conditions can
regularly eat any nuts except peanuts and walnuts.

Peanuts—particularly the redskin, which is a raw peanut
with its magenta-coloured inner skin still in place—contain
vitamin C in the skin but not in the nut itself. Vitamin C is
not usually found in nuts at all, but then the peanut is not a
nut: it's a legume. Nevertheless, peanuts are generally found
amongst the nut products, so we shall discuss them here. The
peanut plant grows as a legume, the fruiting stems diving
down into the ground and producing the 'nuts' on the end of
these stems and below the surface.

The hulls of walnuts, including the papery-thin partitions
between the segments of the nut, are used in herbal medicine,
and they are valuable in treating many diseases of the bowel.

The meal or coarse flour made from ground-up nuts is
much higher in mineral, fat and protein content than flour
made from grain. In almost any dish you make, either sweet
or savoury, you can include a nut meal and so add to the
protein content of the dish in an easily digestible manner.
Ground-up almond is often called marzipan, although mar-

zipan sold as such is not always purely made from almonds but may have additives such as cornflour in it. The pure almond meal has been used for festive cake and sweet dishes from earliest recorded times. The Romans ate nut meal, and the Mesopotamians, and the Chinese; and primitive cultures everywhere have always relied on fruiting nut-trees for a large portion of their protein. Maybe they didn't call it protein or analyse what they were eating, but they knew they felt better with it than without it.

What nuts are most suitable for your physical make-up and dietary needs? To decide this you need to know how they differ. The nuts lowest in carbohydrate content are almonds and pecans and brazils, with walnuts not far behind. The highest in carbohydrate concentration are the cashew nuts. If you are eating nuts and putting on weight, don't, whatever you do, stop eating all the varieties of nut; just stop eating cashews and perhaps peanuts, and go back to almonds and brazils and walnuts. The tiny inside kernels of a particular species of pine tree are sold commercially as pine nuts, and these are highest in protein value, weight for weight, of any nut generally available. Peanuts come a close second, then cashew nuts follow. There is much more fat in cashews, about two and a half times as much as in almonds. All nuts are high in calories compared with other foods—and they are full nutritional calories, not the empty ones of some starches and sugars—so that our energy will return if we nibble raw nuts when our vim and vigour starts to slip during the day.

It is not wise to eat nuts last thing at night, for they do take a long time to digest and your stomach will still be working away when you want it to be relaxed so that you can dream in peace. Many nuts are unbalanced in their mineral content, depending on where they grow. There is the pistachio nut whose potassium content is enormous, but its sodium for counterbalancing is not sufficient to make it a good source of these two minerals by itself. So you have to do the balancing yourself; and I suggest serving pistachios with yoghurt as a delectable dessert, knowing that yoghurt has a very high sodium level. The pistachio nut doubtless grew first in areas where the local inhabitants had sufficient sodium in their diet; for Nature can be trusted to provide the correct nutritional plants for each climate and area and type of people. The trouble starts when we import foodstuffs from vastly different cultures and try to adapt them to our own.

All the nut varieties have a very high iron content, and all have a tiny trace of copper to help the assimilation of the iron. All nuts are lower in vitamins than most food groups, so you are not eating them for vitamin content but for mineral, protein, and vegetable fat. The almond-tree in your garden with the delightful white flowers is not a true edible almond but produces nuts only of the bitter almond variety, which can be dangerously high in hydrocyanic acid. The commercial variety is the sweet almond, which has pink flowers; and if you live in a suitable nut-growing climate you can have several trees so that cross-pollination by the bees will fertilise the blossoms and give you a good crop. Most nuts are high in phosphorus and in the B-group vitamins we have mentioned; so they can benefit your nervous system.

Here is an interesting snippet for gardeners: save all your walnut shells, including the partitions between the nut segments if you can, and smash them with a hammer in a sacking bag, or pulverise them any way you know how. Now add the crushed shells to your compost heap. This makes a compost entirely suitable for propagating cuttings, and the cutting will have not only the same quality as the parent plant but an improved quality of flower and fruit. Why this should be so, I do not know, but it is possible that crushed walnut hulls have a genetic influence in retaining and improving the qualities of plants. I've had very good results, too, from sowing seeds in such a walnut-hull-enriched compost. It appears to have something to do with the fixing of the genetic type so that it retains its best and most vigorous qualities.

And what about peanut butter? It has been said to add to

sexual vigour and, though the manufacturers may have had a hand in spreading this story, there are one or two facts that could point to such a conclusion. Peanuts contain the trace element zinc, and this element has recently been named as a possible factor in determining fertility or infertility. It is true that a total lack of zinc in the diet can produce sterility in laboratory animals, but it is doubtful whether zinc alone is the culprit. So if you lack zinc eating peanuts may help you. If peanut butter separates into oil on the top and a thick, rather dried mass in the bottom of the jar, you can rest assured that it has been untampered with and retains much more of its natural condition than if it is homogeneous in texture all the way through. Hydrogenated oils can be added to it to emulsify it so that it will stay in a uniform consistency; but this means that you are getting hydrogenated fats, which are totally useless and possibly harmful.

Nuts are certainly not a complete replacement for protein from other sources; but they are an uncomplicated and easily obtained addition that will keep much longer than many other types of protein food. The body needs protein to rebuild all those cells that are constantly wearing out or are killed off by disease, and nuts can play an important part in ensuring that your protein intake is sufficient.

Legumes

The term legume covers beans, both fresh and dried, and peas and lentils (as well as peanuts), and these foods can be a hunger-satisfying substitute for protein from animal sources. To vary your protein intake, have bean dishes regularly. They are not only versatile but filling; and for people adjusting to a vegetarian-type diet they can allay hunger and banish the feeling of emptiness.

Beans and peas contain vitamin C when they are fresh, and in a dried state they are still good sources of the B-group vitamins, and very high in iron content. Primitive peoples include beans both dried and fresh in the diet to fill the protein needs when sources of animal protein are scarce.

The different types of legumes vary widely in both protein and vitamin value. Soy beans are the best and most satisfactory food for vegetarians; but when you are tired of them there are dozens of other varieties you can experiment with. There are black-eye beans and red beans; there are brown beans and broad beans. Mung beans, a variety of soy bean, are best when sprouted; and lentils, either orange or brownish-green in colour, can also be sprouted, and are a living source of iron and phosphorus and bromine, the glandular regulator, as well. Lentil soup or lentil flour or lentil sprouts can be included to vary your bean intake and to make hot dishes in the winter-time for appetite satisfaction. I don't know of any vegetarian who can truthfully say that he or she would rather sit down to a cold salad in the dead of winter than a steaming hot bowl of pea soup or a hot bean casserole.

You must soak the dried beans and peas, usually overnight or for quite a few hours before cooking them—but never, never throw away this soaking water, for all your B vitamins are there. If you cook the beans in the soaking water and gradually reduce its volume so that the casserole consistency is not sloshy, you will be getting what is left of your water-soluble vitamins in the juice.

The fresh members of the bean and pea family are quite high sources of vitamin A, and worth including in your diet fresh and young and preferably picked from bushes in your own backyard. These pea plants are so easy to grow and do so much for the soil that they should be the first you try when you start a home vegetable garden.

Grains

Wheat   Wheat and rice are the most widely grown grain foods in the world, and wheat is the best-known grain in Western cultures. Wheat of many different varieties is grown in most parts of the world out of the tropical zone, and its main need for full nutritional value in the seeds is for open sunshine during its growing period. We should try to eat whole-grain products rather than any part of the wheat grain that has been processed. As with every other seed, the husk and the heart are the parts that contain most of the vitamins and minerals; but when the wheatgerm is separated from the wheat grain, and the wheat bran, too, it is only what remains that bakers use in their white-flour-based products. Whole-wheat products are becoming more and more popular as we learn what ghastly mistakes have been made; and wheatgerm, formerly sold only as pig-food, can now be bought as human food without too much bother. But until some brilliant inventor comes up with a method of rolling or cutting whole-wheat grain that handles the whole seed without clogging up the rollers (and upsetting that monster, economic necessity) it is likely that white bread will remain the usual form of bread eaten by the majority of people who still eat bread at all.

It is unfortunate that the steel rollers used in crushing wheat create heat that destroys most of its vitamin content. This is why the health fanatic will not buy anything but stone-ground wholemeal flour, which is fine *if* that stone-ground flour can be proved to be from the whole of the wheat seed. The economic potential of wholemeal flour has been rediscovered to a certain extent by marketers of grain products; but pure, freshly ground wholemeal flour deteriorates quite fast, and an unscrupulous manufacturer may add preservatives and anti-fermenting agents to the flour and still label it 100 per cent wholemeal, which theoretically it still is. If your source of wholemeal bread is a good one, and you are buying loaves that are genuinely made, a loaf will tell you when it's stale by going mouldy within three days in the hot weather and a little longer in the cold weather. If your half-eaten loaf of wholemeal bread goes mouldy, you should praise the Lord (it is free of preservatives) and keep on buying it from the same supplier.

The steel-rolling of flour gives the flour a poor gluten

formation, so extra gluten flour from other sources must be added in order that bread can be made from it at all. White bread that weighs light and has the texture of an open-celled sponge may toast beautifully, but most of what you are eating is holes. The bran of the wheat, the outer husk that is usually milled off, is the mineral storehouse just as much as the wheatgerm in the heart of the seed is. This outer husk is very high in silica, phosphorus and iron and the B-complex vitamins as well, and you're throwing away an enormous and valuable slice of nutritional filling if you don't eat wheat bran sprinkled back on top of your porridge or added to your home-made loaf.

If you have looked at your loaf of wrapped bread and marvelled at the long series of 'vitamin-enriched' properties it has listed, it might pay you to wonder, and perhaps even to ask the manufacturer, what became of the original sources of these vitamins and minerals. The thiamine and riboflavin and niacin and other goodies have been milled out, crushed out, cut out, and thrown out. Only a residual 10 per cent of the original B-group vitamins may be left in the flour after the milling process; and no wonder it has to be 'enriched'.

If only farmers would grow wheat organically again, strong, healthy wheat not prone to the diseases that attack so many crops! Most farmers now believe it is impossible to grow wheat without using superphosphate and other stimulants. But I know of a farmer who has been growing his crops organically for many, many years, and his products are eagerly sought after and analyse like a nutritionist's dream. The protein content is twice as high as that of the best academically grown, synthetically fed crops; the vitamin content is outstanding, particularly the B-group vitamins, and the vitamin E content has soared to levels that have amazed the Department of Agriculture. Bread made commercially from this farmer's flour is a complete meal in one or two slices: it is baked with care and dedication and knowledge of the properties of grain.

Oats The grains of oats contain a tremendous amount of

iron, with its copper trace catalyst, and of calcium, much more than is found in wheat or even in rice. My favourite grain is oats: I eat a large plateful of it each morning; hot and steaming in a porridge in winter, and cold and sustaining in a muesli in summer. It provides me with energy and protein content—very high for a grain product—and phosphorus for the nervous system; and vitamin E and the B group are there in correct balance as well. Oats can also be overprocessed before it gets to you, so that the quick-cooking type may have only half the nutritional value of its slower-to-cook whole type. Even the whole oats may be lower in gluten content now than the rolled oats that used to be soaked on the kitchen table overnight and then cooked for a long and tedious stirring-time the next morning: the present-day cutting method produces some heat that breaks down the seed, making the cooking time for oats considerably less. I don't soak my oats, and I cook them for minutes only, and never to the point where they are jelly-like. For maximum nutritional value, there should be whole chewy pieces of the grain all through a good porridge, and the less you cook a grain, the more vitamin B it retains.

Corn   It is the same with corn. Much of it, grown in various parts of the world, is used to make alcoholic drinks, but the percentage left to us as a vegetable grain food is processed as wheat and oats are, reducing its nutritional value. The eliminating from corn of much of the vitamin B content in processing led to large-scale outbreaks of pellagra all over the world before the precipitating cause was traced: the stripping of much of the worth from grains in the milling process. This was the cause (as was the milling of the outer husk from the whole rice grain much later on) of world-wide symptoms of everything from pellagra itself to much milder forms of B-vitamin deficiency, such as depression and fatigue. It is sobering to recall that in the midst of all this nutritional starvation the Great Depression began: perhaps if we had never milled the goodness out of grains it would not have happened.

Whole corn contains a 'germ' and a husk as other grains do, and when this is milled out to make corn oil, the splitting-up of the whole food leaves a much inferior 'refined' end-product. About one-fifth of the protein of the corn grain is found in the germ or heart or kernel of each grain. The corn oil that is taken from the kernel is a rich source of linoleic acid, which has a big role to play in the assimilation of fats. Although all grain products are not completely blessed with the full range of amino-acids, the whole grain is still a far better food than the unbalanced product you are likely to buy.

Those packaged ears of corn you can get from your supermarket, wrapped in plastic and sealed off 'hygienically', can be about good enough to throw into your compost bin. Corn deteriorates so fast after it leaves the parent plant that it is better either to grow your own or to go to wholesale markets where it is brought in from the farms that morning. If you grow corn, a row or two in your backyard, and you dip those ripened ears straight from the plant into a pot of boiling water until they are just heated sufficiently for you to enjoy, you are really eating corn; or you can nibble your way around an ear of corn fresh from the stalk without cooking it at all, and its floury soft sweetness will astonish you with the flavour of what corn can be. There is vitamin C in corn, too, and this, of course, is one of the first casualties in cooking; vitamin A is also there, and a lot of it, too. Containing almost every mineral and every vitamin, corn is about the most balanced of all grains.

Some foods become more easily digestible if used with other foods: a slice of pineapple on a grilled steak, for instance, so that before it even hits your stomach the meat protein is already being digested by the enzyme material in the pineapple. Putting two foods together, one with an excess amount of some mineral or vitamin and the other with a deficiency, can produce a balanced nutritional pattern. Without the aid of scientific research, primitive peoples found that some foods needed other foods eaten with them to produce a good nutritional result; they found, for example, that the corn kernel did much more for them digestively and nutritionally if it was cooked in lime-water first. Corn cobs were sometimes burnt and the ashes added to food—a mineral supplement taken without laboratory analysis.

Corn muffins and corn bread,. corn patties and corn vegetable casseroles and hotpots, corn salads and corn on the cob—these are all good food. The best method of preserving any corn cobs you cannot eat as fast as they become ripe is to freeze them immediately after picking.

Millet and Rye Millet is a grain much used in Slavic and Asian countries as a source of protein with a low carbohydrate level. Russian athletes train on a diet in which millet is the main grain food, since it gives energy without being fattening. The protein of millet is a simple one and easily digested; its amino-acid count is high, making it a good source of protein.

Rye is often condemned because of its acid-forming properties; but any of the grains are acid-forming in the body. I believe that arthritic people should eat grain foods for the high B-vitamin content, to keep the nervous system functioning well and to help overcome the pain that goes with arthritic crippling: but they must also eat the alkaline-forming foods to balance those acid-forming seeds. The foods with alkaline-forming properties are those high in sodium and potassium, in calcium, magnesium and iron. Check through the lists of these foods in the minerals chapter to find how best to balance your intake.

Rice Some people can live entirely on a diet of brown rice, and it is the staple food in all the 'Eastern' countries where it grows. The polishing and refining of rice to make it white and 'pure' seems to have no justification; and, like many other naturopaths, I'm inclined to blame Louis Pasteur and the antisepsis that was so valuable in other fields: to make the

rice clean, and therefore good for us, contaminating substances had to be removed. Stripping the rice grain of its
seven outer layers of bran and getting rid of the germ of the
rice in the polishing and refining process, means losing most
of the fats, proteins, minerals and vitamins in the grain.
Taking away this protective outer layer means eliminating
about 15 per cent of the protein, about 85 per cent of the fats,
almost 90 per cent of the calcium, and somewhere between
55 and 80 per cent of the B vitamins.

And so the nutritional value of rice was lost, and the world
began to learn how the lack of B-group vitamins could produce the disease called beri-beri. Native peoples in Eastern
countries who changed from a diet of brown to white rice
suffered from this disease, and epidemics of it raged without
any cause then known—until a simple accident discovered
that all symptoms of beri-beri disappeared when brown rice
was reintroduced.

It is true that white rice cooks faster, but it is only a mess of
starch with most of the original nutriment lacking. It takes
a little longer to cook brown rice; and you must cook it so
that all the water is absorbed, so that every trace of its
valuable B vitamins can be retained. Whole rice, nutty-
flavoured and rich in minerals and vitamins, gives you the full
count of amino-acids you need to process any other protein
foods you are eating with it. You may notice when you buy
brown rice that some of the grains are green, and it has been
found that the rice keeps better and has a more 'living' quality
if about three grains in every hundred are green. It is possible
to store such rice for somewhere between twelve months and
five years if necessary, without losing any of its value, if it is
properly dried. It is a good food, needing little care or attention after it is harvested and dried, so long as it is kept away
from weevils—but we must be wary again of economic
necessity, which may have insinuated insecticides into stored
rice.

In some countries white rice, being recognised as of little

nutritional value, is being 'enriched'. Commercialism again
—taking almost all the nutrition out at one end, making it
synthetically, and putting it back at the other end: the white
rice being artificially coated with various substances to attempt to give it back its food value without damaging its
'pure' state.

I use brown rice every other day in either sweet or savoury
dishes, because it is a balanced food, because it is easy to cook
and can be put aside, and because it is readily available all
the year round and not expensive to buy. What we save on
this simple way to good nutrition we can spend on some
luxury such as an avocado or strawberries without feeling
guilty. Rice blends with any other flavour whatsoever. You
can add any spice or herb to it, you can add honey, you can
add cut-up fruit, you can cover it with sauce, you can eat it
simply with a fork, and you can eat a lot of it without its
making you feel overloaded, so that there is good hunger
satisfaction.

Remember, I am speaking of brown rice, the only rice
worth talking about. You can please yourselves as to whether
you use long-grain rice or short-grain or Basmati or any
other variety; and if you have a passion for cleanliness you
can wash that brown rice several times *before* cooking.

The Macrobiotic Diet

The macrobiotic type of diet—the diet that aims to use food
in a more spiritual context to help us to grow in more ways
than just physically—is based on the eating of grain products.
While I believe that any diet balanced with thought and care
can be excellent for many people, I know from experience
with patients that a theoretically good diet is not always one
that works well. It is easier to handle a macrobiotic-type diet
physically if you are of an Eastern race than it is if you are
white and Westernly civilised. Deaths and ill-health have
been caused in young Western people who, in search of a
better way of living, have dived into an ideally 'good' diet

without studying whether it was good for *them*. In one sense it is true to say that we are what we eat; and it is true that food is usually of major importance when we are advising or treating a *whole* person. Unless your physical body is healthy, your mind is not entirely free to be healthy, nor is your nervous system calm enough to let you meditate or contemplate or learn to discover any truths you may be seeking. Although I regard the body as just a vehicle in which to drive around in this world, it makes the journey more pleasant and easier if the vehicle is in A-1 condition, if you can do what you wish to do without being limited by your physical state. What a waste of life to spend years in trying to rid your mind of the pain of rheumatism or your chest muscles of the spasms of asthma when the basic corrective measures can be so simply taken by giving thought to your body's daily needs! What a total wicked waste of good living-time!

SUGAR

So far we have mentioned foods that most nutritionists regard as primary food sources. Now we must talk of a substance that has only comparatively recently come onto the world-diet scene, and that has never been a food in any earlier civilisation than our own.

White sugar is unquestionably a bad food, and although we are constantly confronted with what harm it has done, or what harm it can do, we take no steps to refuse to eat it. White sugar, refined sugar, is taken out of the sugar cane or the sugar beet and sold on its own. It is one of the items regarded as basic in the economy in most Western civilisations; it is included in cost-of-living indexes; and it is one of the greatest turnover articles on supermarket shelves. White sugar is an imitation of something else. What is it an imitation of, and why do we crave it—even if we *do* know what it can do to us?

The craving for sweet things is a part of man's metabolism,

and so it has always been. Sweetmeats or confections have always been seen as something special and rewarding to the body; but the items of which these sweet foods used to be made were dried fruits, like dates and figs, and honey; confections whipped up from dairy products with eggs and milk added to fresh fruit as the sweetening agent; and the tastes of various vegetables, roots and flowers that could be processed using honey. Such foods became special treats to the palate. Why does the human organism crave sweetness? Most animals do not—neither do fishes nor birds, except honey-eating birds. We must look to Nature again: and we learn that vitamins and minerals in their natural form taste sweet. Nature has endowed us with a selective mechanism that tells us what is good for us or what we need; but this mechanism can be fooled by anything that tastes sweet. The increased craving for sweet foods is a basic search after lost vitamins and minerals; and the ill-health that can result from excessive consumption of refined sugar could be Nature's way of telling us we are on the wrong track.

Natural sweet-tasting foods usually have the correct balance of other food nutrients as well as carbohydrates, which are the starches and sugars. Carbohydrates in some form are a must in anyone's diet; they create the energy that enables our physical body to move about and grow and do work and relax. We must have carbohydrates, and the more energy we use the more energy-producing foods we must eat; but these should be selected in accordance with our lifestyle and our body's metabolism. In a healthy body about 70 per cent of all fuel we take in each day is changed into energy; the other 30 per cent is used for building up new cells, repairing damaged old cells, and replacing dead cells. We need this fuel, yes; but from which foods is our daily intake best obtained? Did you know that ripe dates contain between 35 and 75 per cent of *real* sugar, total sugar, complete sugar? Did you know that a pound (454 grams) of grapes can give you four hundred calories of pure sugar energy? The foods that are high in pure carbohydrate energy are corn, beans, potatoes, rice, bananas, and dried fruits; and the body easily converts the carbohydrate found here as starch and sugar combined into the sugars that give energy.

Vast quantities of white sugar are consumed in modern Western society, not only in the form of the white granules in the sugar-basin, but in prepared and processed foods. The whole of civilised humanity has now acquired such an excessive taste for sugar that more and more of it is needed before it can be tasted at all. You might say that those packed bags of 'pure' white refined sugar are selling us a taste—a taste plus empty calories.

Theoretically, 454 grams (a pound) of sugar give you about 1 800 calories of energy; but whether this amount is available to you depends on how your metabolism handles it. The body will use such sugar, if it is available, because it is easier to get a quick reaction from it than to process the fats that are together with it in a natural diet, so that if you give your body loads of white sugar from which to draw its energy it may be storing and retaining any fats you eat. This is the first reason why medical men and nutritionists tell you to cut down on sugar intake to reduce obesity; but it is only a very small part of the obesity picture. If you go off carbohydrates altogether your entire system will be thrown sideways as it tries to obtain energy from protein sources—for it is not used to doing this if you have previously had a heavy carbohydrate diet. White sugar sends glucose in a sudden rush to the liver, which stores as much of it as it can; but if too much sugar is taken the liver protests violently and throws the sugar out again in surrounding globules of fat that are deposited in areas where muscles do not normally work hard and therefore do not get rid of the accumulated fat in the tissues. One of the first areas to suffer is the stomach. Abdominal muscles sag and their tone becomes flaccid. Thigh muscles, atrophied from lack of walking and physical exercise, feel it next.

People who lead a sedentary life and do little or no physical work other than stepping from the car into the office or from the kitchen to the television set, are storing up trouble and are most likely fat. If this type of person drinks a lot of alcohol as well he is delivering a massive assault on his body's storage systems, which can be constantly overloaded. Obesity results. Then he goes on a crash diet of reducing carbo-hydrates of every type, and he has no energy and feels terrible and stops the diet. The ever-decreasing circles he is running around in send him finally to an earlier demise or a pattern of ill-health that can make the rest of his life a sad apology for what life should be. As well as overloading the liver, the massive intake of white sugar overloads the pancreas, the organ that contains the vital sugar-processing substances. An overloaded pancreas means more trouble still—perhaps not diabetes, but possibly an over-activity of the pancreas as it tries to process all that rubbish, leaving a low blood-sugar pattern instead. Many low blood-sugar symptoms are caused in this manner.

I believe that the health of the world is deteriorating faster because of white sugar than from any other single cause. It is not possible to stop a world-wide multi-million-dollar industry by stating that white sugar is harmful, that it is causing disease and ill-health at a soaring rate, costing untold millions in medical care. But surely it should not be impossible to persuade (or legally compel) the executives of these international organisations to turn their gigantic manufac-turing capacity to something that is of value in nutrition? Why not sell the whole sugar, just as it comes from cane and beet? It is in the molasses, the black product that is removed to leave the pure white crystals, that all your food value lies! If sugar was sold as the *complete* product it can be, with its high balanced content of minerals and vitamins, and its value for energy and nutritional compactness, what a product we would have and what a healthy set of earth-dwellers we might all be again! If the housewife can be educated to the

point where she has facts at her command—and this I feel
is an area where the education system has ignored its young
citizens' training—perhaps economic pressure, that monster,
may be turned into a friendly behemoth that will force sugar
manufacturers to sell us the whole thing, and only the whole
thing. Small amounts of black sugar, the nearest thing (after
processing) to the whole sugar, are marketed; but there is
no publicity, no educational information, to boost the sales
of it in preference to white sugar.

Children at school ought to be taught and trained to
know what foods to eat, how foods interact, what a good food
is, and how its processing and preparation can change its
properties nutritionally. The quality of their lives is determined by nutrition. Yet people who are concerned about the
quality or the content of foods are usually branded as cranks.
Many now-famous nutritionists who have stood up for factual
investigation into the quality of the food we eat have been
named as scaremongers trying to undermine the public's
confidence, and even prosecuted by the manufacturers. Now,
in many advanced countries, the contents of processed food
packets must be listed on the label of the product; and this
is as it should be. The world-wide slump in health in civilised
countries during the last two generations is of a magnitude
to make it a prime focus of investigation: and the stress of
modern life, so often blamed, is not the only cause. Do you
know of anyone in your immediate circle of family and
friends who feels absolutely and totally healthy? Do you
know anyone who feels wonderfully well and happy and full
of life and vitality and health? Have you ever asked, 'If not,
why not?' Perhaps you will ask now. If you cease to buy
products you feel are not 'good' food, the food industry may
learn a new sense of responsibility as the profits go down.

Many cases have been recorded of sufferers from allergies
or arthritis who have had no further problems with the
disease when all sugar of the white variety has been eliminated
from their diet. In a strong solution, sugar irritates internal

tissues. It is an artificial, isolated substance that has become an absolute necessity for us before our taste buds can face any form of processed food. You know now that B-group vitamins are needed to handle carbohydrates; and there are absolutely no B-group vitamins left in white sugar. So there is, in eating white sugar, a massive carbohydrate intake without the substances present to control and process it. If you were eating whole sugar (still with the molasses in it) you would be getting an adequate intake of B-group vitamins to handle the heavy carbohydrate load. If you were eating whole sugar you would be getting only about half as many calories by weight portion; but you would be getting whole or full calories, and you would still be getting minerals as well as vitamins. In equal portions by weight you would get 258 times more calcium in whole sugar than in white sugar; and you would get 3 000 times as much potassium.

White sugar is 'refined'; it is 'pure'—terms that apparently mean 'good' to the housewife. Whole sugar is coarse, it's dark in colour, it's 'unrefined'—not good enough for civilised people. Just as wheatgerm was fed to farm animals (it's now fed to humans, too), molasses is sold separately as food for cattle—which is all to the good in making our grazing herds healthier. It's high time we went back to the good earth and her whole products. Once you've used honey or black sugar to sweeten your food you will find your stomach rebelling at the chemicalised taste of white sugar.

Some say that any form of sugar as such is bad for you. If you are getting sufficient vitamin and mineral intake from other sources your need for any form of extra sugar will certainly be less; but it is difficult to rid yourself quickly of the acquired habits of the last two generations. It *is* possible to give up smoking immediately; it *is* possible to go straight off any extra sugars and obtain them only from your food sources: but bodies are not built to be switched on and switched off quite as fast as this. You can do without sugar less traumatically by going from white sugar to raw sugar, then to black sugar, in gradual steps, so that your body can accustom itself to the new pattern.

The sugar you need for your energy can be obtained from simple foodstuffs. Glucose, also called dextrose, is the sugar found in grapes and has the same composition as blood sugar: one good reason why a grape-fast programme can be a good thing for the bloodstream, to normalise it. Fructose is the type of sugar found in fruits and vegetables, and this natural sugar is quite easy for the body to process. Lactose is the sugar found in milk, and this changes to galactose and glucose through the body metabolism. Sucrose is just the chemical name for white sugar, and is one of the constituents of glucose and fructose. Maltose is a grain sugar developed during the malting process; and cellulose is the type of sugar found in fibrous material in the diet, which is almost totally undigested by humans but gives bulk and acts as a sweeping-through agent, physically, as the food works its way through the stomach, small intestine, and large intestine. Inulin is a type of sugar found in all the members of the onion family, and in varying quantities in many herbs. If you are obese and you wish to lose weight by eating foods that have a low carbohydrate value, your best bets here are carrots and peppers, radishes and cauliflower; pumpkin, too, is low in energy value. These foods give you much of the vitamin and mineral requirements needed to wash that clogged-up system of yours clean, and repair its overweight condition.

Once you decide you can do without white sugar strange and wonderful things happen to your taste buds. Just as you find when you reduce the salt, you begin to appreciate the real taste of things: you will recover or discover the faculty for finding sweetness in natural sources. Would you ever sprinkle white sugar on an orange before you ate it? Of course not, it's sweet enough already. It's not easy to convince a husband that that strange taste to his coffee or tea is not poison, just a lack of it; or to tell a child that the new less-sweet taste is better for him. It takes time and patience, but it can be done. The body accustomed to white sugar may experience a state of change that is anything but comfortable; a too-sudden change will throw it temporarily into disarray. But it is such an easy-going, adjustable, long-suffering organism that it will soon acclimatise itself—and you will find that banishing white sugar from your life has been well worth the brief discomfort.

As an aside, insects appear to be attracted to the blood of people who eat sugar excessively, or whose carbohydrate is not being processed correctly. Primitive races are known to vary their food so that when insect time comes round their blood is not appetising to biting insects at all. Think about this if you are particularly vulnerable to mosquitoes, and see whether they find you less delectable when you have cut out those three and four teaspoons of white sugar you normally add to your coffee and tea.

To sum up, people appear to get sicker and sicker as they eat more white sugar and more white flour—the clean, germ-free substances from which the real food value has been removed. There's nothing wrong with anything that looks dark in colour when it's related to natural food. It is the darkest and most heavily coloured fruits and vegetables that contain the highest mineral content, and even from fruit to fruit on the same tree or from flower to flower on the same vine, those with the darkest colour are those with the greatest inherent vitality. The darker the food the better; and when we eat white foods (preferably *not* white rice or white flour or white sugar) such as parsnip and turnip, or the white flesh of the potato, we should balance this by eating a darker food with it: potatoes and, say, carrots; raisins and dates to eat with the whiter flesh of nuts; the dark part of the sugar to eat together with the white; and the darker heart of the wheat and outer bran husk to eat with the residue of white flour. If you only want to go half-way in the health rules, refusing to subject your will-power to any major change, and adhering to the customary white bread, white flour, white sugar, you can at least supplement all the negative things you are eating with a positive intake of counterbalancing or controlling food.

TOBACCO

We know that tobacco is bad for us, that smoking can be a health hazard; but people continue to smoke. The best way, in my opinion, to defeat the tobacco habit is to build up the general health and happiness of the person concerned. Many who find real pleasure in smoking won't agree with me but I believe that anyone with a healthy, happy, contented mind in a healthy body has not much need to smoke tobacco, and that if smoking becomes compulsive and excessive it is a symptom of illness. When a patient comes into my consulting-room and says, 'I want you to give me some herb to stop me smoking', my first answer, if he is that sort of person, is often, 'Well, I can give you a herb that can make you feel so ill that you will not have time to smoke in between trips to the lavatory; or I can give you another herb that can help you to sleep for twenty-four hours each day; or I can give you yet another herb that may kill you off altogether, and you will have no further opportunity to smoke.' Then I tell him that there is no herb on earth which, *per se*, will stop him smoking. All I can do is to help his body to be healthy and perhaps change his outlook a little so that he no longer has such a need to smoke. I have found that once the nervous system of the patient is sufficiently restored to a state of positive health, the need to smoke lessens to the point where it is scarcely there at all.

Smoking releases adrenalin into the system, and every cigarette can give you a little lift. But it also releases your stores of vitamin A from your liver into your bloodstream, and it overpowers altogether your B-complex vitamins: you're left with your nervous system in shreds, your liver playing up, your eyes deteriorating, and yourself feeling so rotten

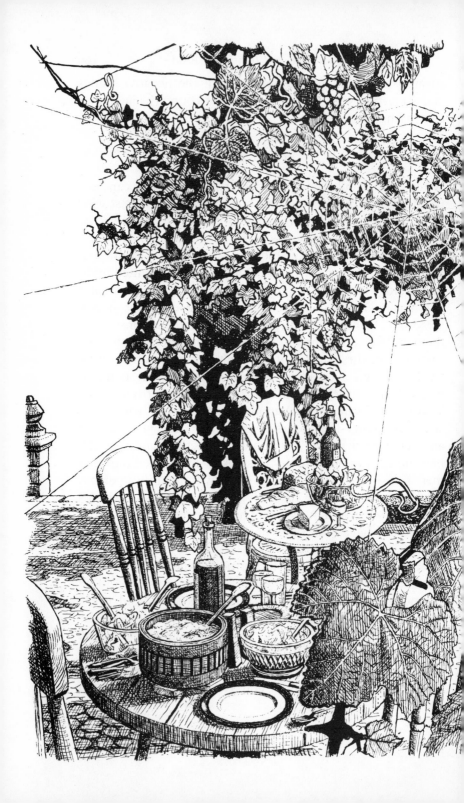

that you reach for another cigarette to make you feel better. Your vitamin C stores are shattered by smoking; and unless you eat a pile of oranges after each cigarette, or a bunch of parsley, or a bag of blackcurrants every day to counteract this effect, you can find that your resistance to disease drops disastrously. The only piece of advice I can give you on smoking as a habit you would like to cut down on, and can't, is to improve the state of your general health. If you learn how to better your state of health and well-being, your smoking habits will change, as will everything else.

ALCOHOL

Intoxication as an escape from our own and the world's troubles has always been with us and will always be. Getting drunk is a habit far more ancient than smoking tobacco. When the ills of the world overpower us, when our personal pressures and tensions mount, we look for oblivion, for a means of escaping for a while. We may get drunk on beer or mead or saki or anything else based on alcohol that takes our fancy, suits our way of living, or fits our pocket. There are other ways of escaping or smoothing out the tension; but, for some, alcohol is it.

The home-made wines of earlier times must have been good beverages indeed, made from fresh herbs and vegetables and fruits and naturally fermented: to be drunk by the wineglassful dose that is often still prescribed in medicinal doses in herbal medicine manuals. Indeed, this is what such wines were—medicinal supplements to provide fluid and the goodness of natural vitamins and minerals in a form in which it could be stored. Wines are no longer drunk only in the area in which they were grown: they are shipped all over the world and changes have had to be made, for this purpose, in the traditional methods of making and storing them. Many of these changes are foreign to the natural fermenting of natural products, the wines having to be artificially strengthened to retain their character under such conditions. Beer produced commercially suffers in the same way, and the distilling of spirits remains one of the last strongholds where an almost pure quality of vegetable product can be obtained, depending on the purity of the water added.

Making alcoholic beverages involves the changing of the basic food used by introducing outside organisms and processes. Whether these organisms are good or bad for the system depends on their quality in the first place. One could say that the very yeast that gives you such a multitude of goodness in its vitamin content is now present working on grapes or cowslips or ginger or rye or apples to break them down into an altogether different biochemical arrangement. Alcohol is perhaps like any other edible substance: good quality and simple forms of processing can give you a product that has a place in a *balanced* form in your diet if you like it. Teetotallers, of course, won't approve of my saying this. But I'll give two examples showing how much health and habit depend on temperament and circumstance.

I had been vainly trying for many months to talk some sense into an arthritic patient who refused to help herself. She was getting no better, and while I was counselling her earnestly one day she suddenly changed the subject: 'I want to bring my husband along to see you so that you can stop him drinking.' I raised an eyebrow, but along her husband came, looking very uncomfortable. I asked him how much he drank. 'One small brandy before dinner and one small brandy before bed,' he answered. 'Yes,' I said, 'what else?' 'That's all,' he answered. I roared with laughter, looked him straight in the eye and said, 'If I had your wife to come home to I'd have *ten* brandies and then not come home at all!' This man's two brandies per night were not only keeping him sane and more relaxed, but keeping the domestic situation under some sort of control. And his wife later confirmed that he never exceeded this quantity. His outlook on life was gentle and soundly balanced in view of the circumstances. He was neither overweight nor unhealthy. The *whole* man was in a good state of balance.

A much younger patient arrived in an extremely distraught state, having rushed straight from work, missed connections, gone to the wrong address. He was now a quivering, frustrated mess, who nervously lighted a cigarette and said, 'God, I need a drink! I can't think at this time of day until I've had a good stiff whisky.' This man showed a state of thorough *imbalance*. He had no self-confidence, no competence in his job. He was fighting to maintain a precarious position in a competitive situation and boosted himself at every stress point with alcohol. His alcohol intake was on the increase every day, and his health was deteriorating at an alarming rate. He had ulcers, his blood pressure went up and down, he was constipated, overweight and miserable. I said, 'Before I can do anything for you, you must stop drinking—and as soon as possible.' Then we talked. Why did he drink so much? He was in the wrong job, hating every minute of it; but he had an ambitious wife. I am not a marriage-guidance counsellor or a psychologist or a psychiatrist; but for his health's sake I said, 'You must either leave your job or your wife. If you don't stop drinking your health is going to become more of a problem than both of these other things put together.' His blood pressure was emotionally triggered as well as complicated by the blood-sugar levels affected by the alcohol. The job stress was the prime cause of the drinking; he would now leave that job and tell his wife why; and he would take whatever consequences there might be. His health would benefit, and so he would be able organise his life much better. All this he worked out for himself.

And four years later that man came into my surgery as he passed through Sydney, a beaming, lean, tanned figure I did not recognise until he told me his name. He was working freelance, as his own boss, on a non-competitive type of practical work he had always loved. His wife had turned up trumps and had given him her support, telling him that his health was worth more than any old job. His wife, who had been sitting in the car, then came in, and their beaming faces convinced me that I had no need to ask about his health. As they were leaving, my professional interest made me ask, 'By the way, how's the drinking going?' He laughed. 'Oh, I still get sloshed occasionally, but now it's enjoyable.' His wife leapt to his defence with, 'Only once in a blue moon. We might have dinner with friends and he has a little too much wine. . . . '

Because wine is made from grapes, it somehow seems to be in a different department from the other forms of alcohol. Grapes are a simple whole fruit, and wine, its fermented juice, can be used in a balanced fashion with benefit to health. A glass of wine drunk with a meal can have positive value; too much wine is obviously harmful and can even kill you. But then you can kill yourself by drinking nothing else but cold water in enormous quantities over a long period. Any food or drink taken to excess can unbalance the metabolism. In simple, peasant-type communities, where wines are made from locally grown grapes, there is always a sturdy *vin du pays* that the people (including children) drink as we drink tea and coffee. This type of wine can be beneficial to health as long as it is not over-indulged in, and the pectin it contains can help the digestive processes. Wine is one of the foods found to be highest in life-energy quality; but this applies only to wine that is simply made from good-quality fruits and vegetables. The loaf of bread and jug of wine could in those earlier days have maintained life and health.

Grapes vary in quality more than most other fruits— depending on how they are grown. They must ripen and mature at Nature's pace in soil that suits them. They must be grown on sunny, open slopes where the sun's rays can fall at the correct angle on the ripening fruit. If you have ever wondered why grapes best grow on hillsides, there is a fascinating theory that the grape is actually 'cooked' from both sides by the sun and the earth, the sun's rays hitting the hillside and reflecting back again on the ripening grapes, with heat energy being converted into natural sugars.

You can make your own simple fruit and vegetable wines, using simple methods; and this wine can be drunk by your family. It should be drunk fairly soon after bottling because it has much more life-energy than more sterile wines, which hold their character longer; and it therefore sours more rapidly as it decomposes to become vineger. There are many informative books available on home wine-making, and you could try some of the recipes they give. If you are not a gardener, try the experience of bargaining at the markets early one morning for the fresh products needed to make a good-quality brew.

When you drink a glass of wine with the meal you should feel little or no intoxicating effect; if you drink two or three or ten or twenty you are unbalancing your metabolism, and must take the consequences. If you don't like herb teas, you may prefer to drink herb wines. It can be an absorbing hobby to make your own, blending flavours, steeping and boiling and straining and experimenting in the garage or the laundry; and your newest blending may be a delightful surprise for your family and friends.

FOOD—IS IT GOOD, IS IT BAD, OR IS IT INDIFFERENT?

It is sad that most of the foods in our present Westernised diet are indifferent foods; and maybe that is why we are such indifferent people: not good or bad, but apathetic and chronically tired and bored; maybe not sick but never really well. Any food that has been tampered with since it left its growing medium can be called indifferent, even if its positive values have been replaced by additives and 'enrichments'. Any food that is only a part of a whole food can be called bad food, for it is deliberately unbalanced and more harmful than those packaged, processed, bland, easy, enriched and neutral foods. How stupid of Man to change a balance Nature has placed in a food perfectly in the first place! When the living quality is missing from food, eating it leaves you feeling dissatisfied or unsatisfied; and the foods we must learn to seek out are the ones that can thrust us out of neutral gear and into top, cruising along without effort, with a forward propulsion into good health. Living foods are what we need, foods that are simply grown and freshly gathered just before we eat them.

Even a tiny plot of ground or a sunny balcony full of growing things in pots could be enough to tip the balance between good or indifferent or bad health. Pick your own vegetables five minutes before putting them into the pot or eating them fresh; find a farm where, on your week-end drive, you can pick up eggs laid fresh that morning; try to eat foods produced within a marketable distance of your home. Don't underestimate the power in simple food. And don't prepare the food you are going to eat too early: this can make it indifferent food. Don't shell the nuts, peel the fruit, and soak the vegetables hours before the meal. Seeds, too, deteriorate when they have been crushed into flour for weeks or months before use; and so do fruit juices that have been pressed from the fruit and stored far too long after the first glassful.

The aim with positive or creative eating is to store your food in a whole state, breaking it up to eat only at the last moment. You can grind your own flour from different grains, buying the whole grain and crushing it at the very last moment in a coffee-grinder or wheat-grinder before cooking it or using it raw. Do swapping with other gardeners in your neighbourhood. One may have an enormous mulberry-tree, and you may be able to barter half a dozen cabbages and some oranges to make marmalade for some ripe mulberries. Use the soil, the good earth soil, to create health for you with whatever you grow in it. Let reason and balance and harmony guide you in your return to the natural foodstuffs that will bring you natural health.

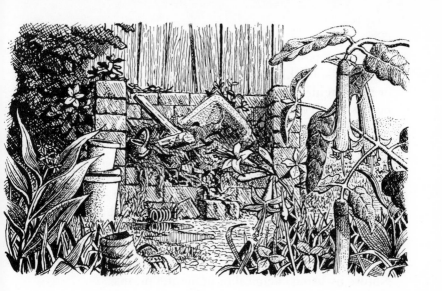

5

Organic Growing

WHAT IS IT?

Have you ever seen a forest that has grown naturally in straight rows of trees spaced equally apart, or of equal height and without vegetation growing underneath? Have you ever seen daffodil bulbs subdivide themselves into neat rows? Would you enjoy sitting on a creek bank in a national park on a warm Sunday afternoon where there were willows spaced out along the bank with mathematical precision, and underneath each willow a gorse bush, and underneath each gorse bush a clump of rushes at the water's edge?

Nature has no straight lines, uses no measuring-sticks, and her plantings are haphazard in the extreme. But Nature's plantings always grow, because the seeds germinate and the roots run only if the natural conditions are favourable. Man rejoices in his small superiority by being able to decide where he wants something to grow, planting seeds and arranging or rearranging his environment to suit himself. Traditionally he has planted in neat rows, in formal square and circular beds primly and symmetrically laid out. But the landscape architects of today are learning from Nature, creating small environments of such beauty and with such skill that they look like Nature's own work. Wanting to have a choice in what he grows, and where and when, man has learnt to organise natural processes. He has also divided his gardening into two broad categories: one copies and concentrates natural growing processes, and this has become known as organic growing; the other tries to improve on and change Nature by using chemical or unnatural means.

I have a strict rule with my herbs and vegetables, and even with my weeds and self-sown wildings: they stay where they grew in the first place. If this means that my terraces are full of self-sown plants after good rains, or the violets creeping across my lawn interfere with what I had planned, then I sit down and contemplate where the plants have put themselves and ask myself whether they know better than I do how to landscape a garden. I struggled for many years with a wild patch near the fence of my previous home, wondering whatever to do with its wandering-jew-covered weed-clumps and rocks and old rubbishy timbers and piles of accumulated refuse bequeathed to me by a previous owner. I gave up the struggle finally, having removed the wandering jew over a few week-ends, and let Nature take over. Within two seasons this rubbish corner was the most delightful spot. Amongst the rubbish had been seeds of hawthorn dropped by the birds, and two small hawthorn-trees grew, one against the fence and one farther forward, and below them the wandering jew had been annihilated by a dense thicket of twining self-sown honeysuckle. Behind this, small fuchsia bushes struggled through from my neighbour's garden towards my sunnier side of the fence, and their fairy ballerina blossoms dropped from the branches onto a thick mat of violets that by some miracle had washed down from farther up the hill in a storm and sown themselves in a perfectly contoured border around the gravel edges of the pathway. Up through this conglomerate mass of exuberance would come a lily bulb struggling through with its white perfumed trumpet heads, or a stand of goldenrod, come from heaven knows where, or some of my favourite wild plants, the plantains, with their spear-shaped rosettes of leaves and their knobbly flower-heads. One year, bursting through the undisturbed vegetation, I had forget-me-nots, which I had never seen before and never saw again at this spot. It was a good lesson in landscaping—to stand back and observe the health of plants growing where and when they found the correct conditions.

In my present home I have a clump of bananas in a mini-patch of semi-tropical warmth in a far corner of the garden, and some stands of wild ginger below them, and a vine of passionfruit climbing in amongst the banana stems and up the fence and off to goodness knows where in my neighbour's property. Right beside this tropical effulgence is growing a plant that theoretically should never grow in such conditions —a pear-tree that sowed itself there and has flourished ever since. Pears prefer a cooler climate, but this one is strong and healthy and content, and growing prodigiously. I have plants I am told need an acid soil and plants I am told need an alkaline soil growing side by side and thriving merrily because they sowed themselves there in the first place.

The berry-bearing trees and shrubs are the star performers in self-sowing, because birds drop the seed after eating the fruit. This type of natural sowing would not happen without the birds; without the natural contours of the land and the rain that washes seed and refuse and compost down; and without the insects to pollinate from flower to flower, from tree to tree and from vegetable to vegetable. And now our insects and birds and the natural drainage of water from high ground are all disappearing: the insects poisoned; the birds gone when their insect food-supply goes; the contours of the land blocked off and rearranged so that drainage water is lost into concrete pipes and does not see the earth again.

The term 'organic' seems to me inappropriate and misleading. Every growing thing. every living thing, is organic; so you cannot have a garden without something organic going on, chemicals or no. It is merely a handy word to differentiate between natural gardening methods and artificially controlled gardening; and it has come to mean growing plants without synthetic fertilisers, without chemical fungus inhibitors, without pesticides, weedicides, soil conditioners, and sprays on foliage and budding fruit. But this only tells half the story and the negative half: organic gardening means *not* doing all those things. To understand and benefit from organic gardening you must take advantage of its *positive* contributions, not only keeping your garden free from synthetic treatments and artificial conditions but using Nature's patterns intelligently to produce healthy plants and prolific crops and disease-free vegetables. If we give ourselves time to observe Nature at work, we can learn and profit a great deal by copying her methods.

The three elemental forces Nature uses are sun, rain and the earth. If any of these three is missing, the other two cannot function alone. Because we are earthbound, let's start with the soil itself.

THE SOIL

Do you really know what the soil is? Have you ever looked closely at a lump of soil? You will find that the particles that compose it are of widely differing natures but all have originally been parted and decomposed and crumbled and chipped away by temperature and by pressure from rock. Here we have our mineral basis of environmental soil conditions. Whatever the original primal rocks were, the soil is now composed of minute particles of it. If you live in a limestone, or shale or sandstone area, the basic nature of your soil will contain originally only the minerals present in the rock from which it came. Each tiny solid particle is further broken down, and further still, until an ideal state of friability is reached, in which the roots of living plants can rest happily and absorb the nutriments that lie between the particles. Soil itself, or the tiny particles of pulverised rock that compose it, would never grow any living thing: the important part of the soil is what lies between the particles. Here we find the microscopic life with which the soil teems and pulses and recreates in the most efficient of all natural perpetual-motion cycles. The organic or living matter that has died returns, at its death, in some fashion to the soil. From this dead fibre of leaves and bark and fruits, of flowers and seed-heads and grass roots and weeds, comes the germ of new life as it is broken down by soil bacteria. We all know of the carbon cycle, that animal/plant relationship where the animal eats the plant and then returns to the soil the manure that helps a new plant to grow for the animal to eat. There is an equally vital process going on in the soil where the dead plants are broken down by a multitudinous collection of the most beautiful creatures imaginable when they are seen under a microscope or with a powerful magnifying glass: the earthworms, the fungous and parasitic animals, the bacteria, and the microscopic soil life of the kind you see teeming inside your compost heap when you take that first shovelful to put on your garden.

Some time ago I showed my students two samples of soil from the same garden: one I had taken originally after I moved here, and one I took some four years later after using natural methods to enhance the soil's fertility. The first sample was a thick reddish clay in which granular soil particles predominated, with little or no humus material and lumps closely adhering to each other, dry and compacted. The other sample almost walked out of its jar to show them! This soil was nearly black in colour, each particle separated one from the other to form a coarse, loose mixture somewhat like the particle size of raw sugar. Amongst all this loose mineral material, trekking about in the blackish-brown mixture, was a teeming horde of soil organisms. We looked at some of these under a microscope, and the beauty and variety of the animals there made my students gasp as they realised what was going on under their feet.

How do you change one type of soil into the other? First you use two qualities with which humanity is endowed to a greater or lesser degree—patience and common sense. If you can put into your soil so much decayed vegetable matter that there is abundant food for all these soil organisms, it stands to reason that you will get better soil according to the amount of decayed material you put into it. When you take as much as you can out of a system, any system, without replacing it at the other end, the system breaks down altogether. The pace of modern absorption requires a faster pace of cultivation, and Science has led us astray in letting us believe we can continuously rob the soil and get away with it. It took many years for the American farming population to realise that the god of Science had let them down in trying to transform Nature using Science alone. Use Nature to aid Nature, and Science to aid Science: The way to control or improve or use or restore a natural system is to use natural means.

Compost

How do you get your soil to change into this rich organic living stew? You can start off in a commonsense way and return to the soil every bit of dead plant material and animal refuse you can. You can do it fast with a mulching machine—such machines now being available in models ranging from household size to an enormous industrial type that can chomp up tree-trunks. You can also do it by saving one small corner of your backyard or one pot-plant-size corner of your balcony for a compost heap. You can construct scientifically proportioned compost bins that will recycle all this waste material in a form you can use; or you can try open-heap composting. One of your sources of compost is the left-over waste from kitchen vegetables and animal remains—the skins of fruits, the pods of peas, any vegetable snippings whatsoever, cooked vegetables left over uneaten on the plate, chop-bones, fish-heads, eggshells, tea-leaves.... I have a square container on my kitchen counter into which goes every bit of re-usable material each day—all the vegetable and animal bits, herb-tea residues, even dead flowers from the vases. Sometimes I add the dust from the carpet-sweeper, but only if it is from a woollen carpet, not a synthetic one: nylon fibres will not break down in compost. Each evening this box is emptied onto my compost heap, and you would be surprised at the bulk of it by the end of the week.

You can become very dedicated to all this, having three compost bins constructed side by side that you fill religiously at one end and turn into the middle and turn again into the end so that you have a rotation of compost materials available. Or you can just throw all your waste vegetable matter in one heap and let time and sun and rain and soil organisms do the work for you in an untidier fashion. In my new graden— new to me, but a well-planted and well-cared-for garden over many years—I found a bonus: at the back, what I thought was a heap of rubbish and old iron, covered over with wandering jew and thick runners of kikuyu grass, turned out to be a pile of rich black compost. Some previous owner had laid it down and not used it, leaving it for me, to blanket all my small transplanted herb treasures: a sweet-smelling, black, rich cover to feed them until they became established.

I could be very detailed about this composting ritual, giving you quantities and amounts and sizes, and a timetable on how often to compost what and when to mulch which; but I firmly believe that this is not the way to successful gardening. Growing things—or, rather, giving growing things the conditions in which they can be healthy and flourish—is an art, not a science. If you don't know when your plants need something you may as well give up being a gardener and take up ten-pin bowling! Just as you know when your family is feeling hungry, or ill, surely you know when a particular shrub is looking seedy, yellow, starved and unhappy or wilting from lack of water or drooping miserably at flowering season instead of bursting with bloom? It's not really a case of what to give it—it's a case of giving it what every plant needs, which is natural organic food.

Trees drop leaves over a short period fast, or bit by bit during the year. There is nowhere else for these leaves to go but onto the ground, where they should be (in natural surroundings) rotted well away by the next season. You will find that Nature works on a seasonal basis almost without exception. Whatever should be available for the plant in its flowering or its maximum-growth period is there, having been started off twelve months earlier. Of course, we must keep our garage floors free of piles of autumn leaves blown in, and our patios swept clean of spent flowers and twigs; but we can do as Nature does by storing all these in the one spot so that the soil bacteria can start to work and a pile can be accumulated and ready for use.

In order to obtain as rich and complete a plant food as naturally possible we must draw from many vegetable sources and use common sense as to what to leave out. Never add fats or oil to compost, or any newspapers that will become compacted and let no air at all through; do not add synthetic clothing materials such as nylon or rayon; and never add polythene bags or wrapping. Cardboard is not too good, either, if it has printing or colour on its surface, since the inks these days are not made with vegetable dyes. Never add plants that are diseased: although the heat generated in the heap should kill most things, some fungous spores may be left surviving in the moisture. Never add kerosene or detergents, and try to keep out any plant waste that has been sprayed with pesticides, for these could kill soil micro-organisms.

Wood—partially rotted—and bark pieces are fine, but don't add old timbers or chips if they have ever been sprayed with creosote.

You must also use common sense so that you do not make the entire compost heap of grass cuttings or beech-leaves or eggshells: mix a little of everything, so that there is a complete balance of all possible nutrients the plants may need. The plants will take whatever they need from the compost and leave the rest for the plant next door or farther along the row.

Many people ask whether it is not courting disaster to add weeds such as couch-grass and kikuyu grass to a compost heap. The answer is always the same: a small amount of anything will not do any harm and it will certainly not re-propagate if you leave it to decompose quickly and if you build the compost heap in the correct manner in the first place. The whole idea of composting is to retain the natural breakdown products within the heap so that they are not left to drain off into the surrounding soil as in Nature, but are retained for more direct use on your garden.

The best size for a compost area has been found to be a bin or a space of approximately 90 centimetres square and 90 centimetres in height (a cubic yard). This bin size is about what you need in a temperate climate to generate sufficient heat at its centre, as the materials decompose and rot away, to ensure that all the plant material is in a broken down, composted state when you want to shovel it over your garden beds. A smaller size than this, even though you have the right materials in it, may not generate sufficient heat—depending, of course, on where it is situated. I have my compost bin with its back to a stone wall where there is shelter from sun and wind, so that heat is retained in the stones from the heap and not dispersed into the air all around. A compost heap, rather than a bin, must be larger than this because it presents more surface to the air and therefore loses heat more rapidly.

It is not absolutely necessary to cover your bin with a close-fitting lid. I cover mine with a wooden slatted lid, so that air and light and a little rain can still penetrate but the sun cannot unduly scorch or the wind unduly dry. How long the compost will take to break down into a usable condition will vary according to the location of your compost bin. I like to use mine while it is still rough and fairly coarse, for I strew it on the surface of the soil, and any small twigs and sticks and pieces of bark and leaves still fibrous and recognisable give a surface mulch, while the more rotted material amongst it all drains happily underneath into the soil. The length of time your bin of compost takes to break down also depends on the season of the year in which you make it: naturally in a humid summer, in a warm corner of your garden, it will go faster than during midwinter, when any heat it generates has to be its own, and heat loss externally is greater.

You can make a small quantity of compost on a balcony if you use an old plastic tub, or a plastic garbage bin with holes cut here and there in the sides, and the bottom removed. Fill the bin with smallish amounts of this and that—even weeds pulled from the footpath if you have no other garden—and put a lid loosely on top. Remember to keep it all moist either from the rain or by your own watering of it every so often. The heat as the sun strikes the plastic container will be quite sufficient to start composting processes in there, and the smaller area of bin would suit the home-unit dweller who has only a pot-plant garden to cater for.

You can make a simple compost bin from a few scrounged bricks or concrete blocks stacked round in a square. This type of bin is easy to disassemble, so that you can get that last rich black shovelful from the bottom. I have to remove only the front part of my bin, which consists of concrete brick sections not too heavy for me to lift but thick enough to retain heat and moisture.

The making of compost needs not only rotting plant and vegetable material but also excreta and a certain amount of soil. The easiest way is to fill your bin with alternate layers 10 to 20 centimetres (4 to 8 inches) deep (depending on the size of the container) first of vegetable material, then a thorough sprinkling of animal manure (either farmyard or stable manure), and finally a layer of good soil to provide some of the first-stage bacteria needed to start decomposition. It is not even necessary to use good soil: you can use thick clayey lumps that will break down and become pulverised by the action of organic and bacterial agents, so that you are doing a double job—correcting the soil as well as making the compost. Build up a bin like this, with layers alternating, until it is full right to the top. Have a container of lime close by, so that you can sprinkle a light handful through as you complete each layer. Lime is essential for composting because it provides such a lot of calcium to keep the bin contents sweet, and it plays a direct role in the breakdown processes too. Following these simple rules, you should have a binful of compost ready for use somewhere between eight and twelve weeks from the time it was filled. There is a faster way, too: several specific herbs added to the compost break the whole thing down in six to eight weeks instead.

Be prepared for the material in the bin to sink as you add each layer. Keep on adding to it, remembering that the material on the bottom will probably rot first—this is where the turning of the bin comes in. I have never found this as necessary as some people say it is; but theoretically it's a good idea to turn the entire contents of the bin from top to bottom once during the composting cycle, or if you have two bins one next to the other, turn the first lot of material into the second one from top to bottom. This will give you an even rate of decomposition, ensuring that the whole heap is in the same state of breakdown. Heat generated to decompose the pile is sufficient to rot away weed seeds and flower seeds and roots of plants. But it is better to keep very fibrous material out of your compost heap, for it breaks down more slowly and you will have an uneven texture. The compost heap, after it is filled up to the top of the bin, should be about as moist as a wrung-out sponge. This is one of the reasons why you must leave spaces here and there for drainage, and I suggest that if you build your compost bin of cement blocks or bricks or hardwood timber, you leave air-vents about 30 centimetres (12 inches) apart to ensure the vital aeration of the heap: otherwise you get compressed, rotten silage that is of no use to anyone and smells quite atrocious. You must provide some form of aeration when you are placing the initial layer on the bottom of the bin, so that any rain-water that does get in, or surplus drainage water as you keep the bin moist, can drain away. Some organic gardeners collect small cans about 7 centimetres (3 inches) in diameter and 3 centimetres (1½ inches) deep and put them open side down to make a floor all over the bottom of the bin, thus providing air and drainage; and as the tins begin to rust away and rot down, they can add iron in minute quantities to the final product. If you don't like the idea of tin cans in amongst your precious organic stuff you can make a thickish floor of twigs and good-size branch stems, all criss-crossed in a mat about 7 centimetres (3 inches) deep.

The whole idea of composting is to use the heat generated by rotting vegetable and animal remains to reduce them to a form in which they can be recycled for the plants you wish to feed. The temperature inside a well-made compost bin can reach somewhere between 48 and 65 degrees Celsius! This temperature should ideally be reached within the first few days of completely filling the bin, and should be somewhere near this even in cooler weather and when the bin is in a semi-sheltered spot. It is not necessary to have the compost bin or heap in full sunshine—in fact, it is better not— although I do like mine against a stone wall to retain the 'cooking heat'. The temperature can be achieved irrespective of the weather if the bin is properly made up of a little of everything with the layer of soil and manures and the sprinkling of lime in between. Keep a container of lime or dolomite handy (lime is calcium carbonate, dolomite is a mixture of calcium carbonate and magnesium carbonate) to keep the bin sweet and the neighbours from complaining, and to deter the odd mouse or rat or possum from raiding the vegetable and food scraps.

Put simply, organic composting is just duplicating the natural conditions every plant is seeking. In the forests and grasslands and mountains, as the trees grew old and fell, as annual plants and weeds died off, a deep carpet of decaying material formed on the surface of the ground. No one came along with fork or hoe, expecting bigger and brighter flowers and heavier crops of fruit and berries—and time allowed the surface treatment to do the job. Amongst this mulch would be found the bones and manure of animals: those that had died returning their entire skeletons and decomposing flesh to the flies and other predators and then indirectly back to the soil, and those still walking around dropping faeces in the form of natural manure. If you can adhere as closely as possible to a natural manner of things you are going to give the plants what they need, in spite of what all those scientific gardening books tell you they must be dosed with. It is not possible to over-compost your garden as it is possible to over-apply synthetic additives; and the more compost the plants receive the more lush and tropical the growth as you imitate the heavy, moist mats of compost found in rainforest areas. The more compost, the more growth of a natural, not a forced, variety; and you never need to worry about 'over-feeding'.

Soil with an adequate compost content (administered in, say, two or three doses each year) and with a natural balance of organic minerals returned to it in the form of dolomite—that great alkaliser of soils—enables you to grow alkaline-loving plants in a native soil that is basically quite acid. Add a ration of blood-and-bone and hair—some type of animal fertiliser containing if possible the bone material and the keratin fibres of hair and skin—so that the valuable potash is not missing from the soil. Bear in mind that the manure from animals is only as nutritious to the soil as the health of the animals from which it came. Poultry manure from battery-housed hens fed with artificial hormone-added chemically filled pellets is certainly nowhere near as good for your garden as the manure from birds that can peck and feed from the earthworms and grasshoppers and green matter and grubs in the backyard garden or poultry run. If only we had sufficient land each so that everyone could keep a cock and half a dozen hens—oh, what vegetables and flowers we would be able to grow and how little time we would have to spend with pesticides and sprays! I am doubly lucky in that the lower portion of my garden was once enclosed for poultry. The grass here grows so lush and thick and the fruit-trees and vegetables I have planted are so healthy and strong and abundant in their harvest that I bless again and again those generations of fowls that ran to and fro underneath. On this section of the garden, and particularly in the lawn, there are earthworm casts a few centimetres apart over the entire area. Synthetic chemicals destroy the earthworm, this guardian of the soil's health.

Earthworms

The earthworm was always considered the lowliest form of animal life, so much so that any sub-standard human being was often referred to as a worm. It is chastening to find that without earthworms none of us would have been able to live on this planet in the first place, for no vegetation could grow and die and re-grow from the products of plant decomposition without the silent underground recycling system perfected by earthworms. It is even more sobering to think that the earthworm is often the last living organism to give its attention to our earthly bodies. This humble creature has no voice and no brain; it has the patience and timing of a computer and the muscular activity of a highly evolved creature, and every decayed piece of vegetation and animal life provides food that is transformed as it passes through the body of the worm into good-quality fertiliser. The animal has calciferous glands that transform the dead material, much as lime or dolomite breaks down dead plant and animal remains. Worms consume large quantities of food as soon as the soil is moist enough to trigger their timing mechanism, and this is one good reason for keeping your garden well watered in dry weather. Earthworms cannot go into action unless sufficient moisture is there.

It is about right to say that the territory underneath a fertile, well-cared-for, well-fed pasture or garden is more densely populated than any overcrowded human civilisation. The weight of earthworms processing waste in the soil is roughly equal to the combined weight of the cattle or sheep grazing on top of an organically grown pasture. Worm-casts contain many nutritious elements that are not found in the soil in which they live and that therefore must have arrived there through the digestive processes of the worm as it recycled dead vegetation and animal life: five times more nitrogen, seven times more phosphate in available form, eleven times more potash and about 40 per cent more humus than was there for the worm to eat in the first place. An astonishingly productive animal to put to work for you in the vegetable patch or rose garden.

Other Soil Inhabitants

Yeasts and moulds and fungi live in the soil too—millions of them. They all break down decaying vegetable and animal matter, and without these below-ground helpers all of civilisation would be covered in rotting accumulations of waste. There is another underground relationship where one class of plants helps another, and this is the mycorrhiza/plant team: this minute organism lives half in the soil and half in the root of the plant, transferring nutriment directly from the soil humus into the root system. Most of our flowering and fruiting plants take part in these relationships, especially when compost is present in quantity.

There are bacteria in the soil, too, living relatives of the same type of 'wog' that invades human cells, and many of them are helpful underground in symbiotic relationships with plants. The commonest and most outstanding example of this relationship with bacteria is in the way leguminous plants of the pea and clover families form nodules on their roots where nitrogen-donating bacteria receive free carbohydrate from the plant. Growing of clovers and lupins and various pea-family crops on poor pasture can result in the equivalent of about 6 tonnes of superphosphate per hectare being deposited in a natural form under the ground, where the roots of the following crop can get into it right from planting time. Think of the saving in money, work, time and worry! Your fertiliser is being spread and dug in for you while you are asleep at night or even far away from your land!

If you haven't any earthworms in your garden you can get them there fast by increasing the humus content of your soil with compost. It is even a good idea for you to have an earthworm or two in house pot-plants, for these benefit from natural growing, too. As a child of five or six, I was given the job of looking after the distribution of earthworms in my parents' garden. I remember digging deep down into rich beds covered with manure mulches to find earthworms to take to a new part of the garden, just designed, where the subsoil had been uncovered and the thick red clay was resisting the efforts of pick and shovel to break it up. I made numerous trips, under instructions from my mother, with a small toy barrow into which I dropped all the earthworms I could dig up from the fertile soil, and these were turned in with manure and compost and vegetable waste and a load of imported topsoil. In two seasons this new garden was the pride of my mother's collection of roses. Shot Silk and Black Boy climbers covered the fence with translucent shell-pink and deep crimson blooms, and the bush roses flourished underneath. The bed was dug only about once a year. The rest of the time it was mulched with compost and lime, and I remember going out to see if my transplanted earthworms had made it. They were there, all right, generations of them, and that hard clay-pan subsoil, broken up by the two years' work of worms and humus, was there no longer.

HERB-ACTIVATED COMPOST

If you grow herbs you should have found by now that compost is the food they enjoy the most; and you can do a lovely bit of ecological recycling here by using some of the herbs to help in making the compost by way of return thanks.

Comfrey

The first and probably most useful herb of all is comfrey, *Symphytum officinale*, which grows in its spinach-like enormous clumps from one season to the next, although it dies right back to the ground in winter in cool or highland areas. This herb, semi-miraculous on the health scene, is most valuable for gardeners, since its leaves when broken down to a jelly-like, rotting state contain approximately the same balance of minerals as are found in horse manure. Comfrey grows and spreads so fast that there will be plenty for all your needs—for your salads, for your skin, for the treatment of burns and cuts and various ailments, *and* for your garden beds and compost heap.

The comfrey plant must be in the open garden where its roots can forage to some depth. The roots go down and down, opening up hard clay-pan soils and providing channels for water to penetrate as they go. Comfrey can be used for draining a soggy section of garden—and the plants will thrive because copious water is necessary for their own growth. Their leaves transpire enormous quantities of water on warm days, and they need plenty of watering in dry seasons, so that the soft leaves do not faint away. But once they are firmly established and their roots are foraging deep down, they can withstand more climatic shocks. Water the leaves as well as the roots of comfrey and you will replace lost moisture more quickly and prevent the leaves drooping and browning.

This wonderful herb, with its long-stemmed fleshy leaves growing so rapidly, can be cut and put in the compost bin each time you add another load of waste material. You can use as much comfrey as you have to spare, but put in at least a dozen leaves for each 8 inches (20 centimetres) in the bin. Comfrey breaks down compost because of a highly complex chain of events that it is not the purpose of this book to describe in technical detail; but its ration of vitamin B_{12} (the vitamin found in organic decaying matter) triggers off and speeds up the decomposition of other vegetation. Comfrey can greatly benefit any plant growing near it, draining the soil, adding nitrogenous compounds as its underneath and outer leaves break down and drop, stirring all the soil organisms into rapid activity with its vitamin B_{12}.

Do not grow comfrey against a hot wall or in an enclosed courtyard where heat can generate in the middle of the day, unless you are prepared to water thoroughly every evening in the hot weather. It must be grown in full sun, yes, but give it some shelter from the worst of the summer heat, preferably with a green wall of other shrubs to absorb the hottest rays of midsummer sun.

It is possible to make a liquid manure from comfrey leaves, but it is faster and simpler to chop up the fresh leaves and lay them about on the surface of the vegetable beds or gardens for a few days until they dry. Then fork them lightly below the surface, where they will become jelly-like and decompose extremely rapidly to provide nearby plants with nitrogen.

Yarrow

The second of the herb plants you can use in composting is yarrow, *Achillea millefolium*. Yarrow has an effect on compost that is truly unbelievable until you see it happen. Just two leaves of yarrow, chopped up coarsely and scattered roughly through a normal-sized bin of compost, have astonishing results. There is no need to place them accurately in any way at all; it is just beneficial to have them there. And if you put more yarrow than this the entire process will go not faster but more slowly! Those two leaves act as a catalyst in the bin, triggering off a natural fermentation process. In about a week's time, when you lift the lid of the bin, you will find that the contents have shrunk approximately by one-third after the yarrow has been introduced: the entire breakdown process has been speeded up. Yarrow used with comfrey can give you organic compost in six to eight weeks.

Camomile

The third herb for use in composting is camomile. High in vegetable calcium, as comfrey is, it helps to banish bad smells from a bin that has not been properly put together or in which the waste material has been wrongly stacked. You can drink camomile tea (which you can buy from your health store), making it as you would a normal pot of tea, putting the little yellow cone centres of the flowers in a teapot and adding boiling water. The pulpy dregs from this strained tea you can then tip into your kitchen waste container and then onto the compost heap. There is still enough calcium left in the camomile pulp to do an efficient job.

Nettles

If you are in a region where stinging nettles grow, thank your lucky stars and use them. Add the entire plant of nettle, chopped up into 7 or so centimetre (3 or 4 inch) lengths, to the compost bin—as much as you like because it is replacing the long-lost heavy iron that has washed down and out of our topsoils over thousands of years. This iron is what no growing thing can get along without, and it must be made available again before the soil can be called truly fertile. You can also boil nettles up as a green vegetable, steaming the young growing tips or adding them to soups and stews as one of the best sources of natural iron. You can plant nettles as a hedge to keep the neighbour's dog at bay, or you can have them growing thickly around newly planted shrubs so that animals will not knock them over. You can try growing stinging nettles in amongst your herbs or under your rose bushes, or in amongst vegetables for an increase in flavour or for better quality and quantity of flowers and fruit. Nettle is a wonderful activator (for people as well as plants), and the very acid that causes the sting of a nettle is the thing that stimulates and feeds the fine hair-roots of a plant, be it tender annual or bushy shrub.

Dandelions

You can also add dandelions to the compost, even the seed-heads, without courting disaster if your bin is properly filled: the heat should kill any such weed seeds, changing them into life-giving humus. Use the tops only of the dandelions as you strip them from formal beds or pathways or cracks in the paving on the terrace, so that the root will be there to go on providing you with more leaves for your next batch of compost. Dandelion leaves provide valuable iron and calcium and have the same sweetening effect as camomile flowers in keeping the compost heap inoffensive.

This is true ecological balancing. The herbs help the compost and the compost helps the herbs, and no outside agents need be introduced or removed. Organic growing can be said to be a process in which humans attempt to copy Nature and apply her methods in a more concentrated form. Random organic gardening gives us the equivalent of natural bushland: intelligently applied organic processes use Nature's good ideas to produce the natural health and growth, the natural flowering and fruiting, of the plants we wish to grow. Nature can afford to take her own time and do her organic gardening over thousands of years: we must condense our gardening to fit our short life-span.

ORGANIC GROWING AIDS

Ash

Those swirls of blue smoke in the autumn when righteous gardeners (and non-gardeners) are burning fallen leaves! Of what use is the by-product, the ash? Many gardeners burn off all their waste material and shovel off loads of black and white ash in all directions, believing it is good nourishment for their plants. This ash works in one major way only: it lightens heavy soils; but as a source of nutrition for plants it is worthless because the potash the ash contains is not in a form in which this necessary element can be absorbed. If you are going to use wood ash at all you should put it, together with other materials, in the compost bin, so that the light, porous particles can be assimilated with the composting material and improve its aeration and texture.

If you have plants in pots, perhaps because you live in a home-unit, you may save your barbecue ashes and use them not as a plant food but as drainage material in the bottom of the pots. Sift the large charcoal pieces out and use a layer of these to provide natural drainage.

Soot

If you are blessed with some form of coal fire, or if you can manage to sweep an odd chimney or two, or if you have a slow-combustion stove and can sweep the vent, you have an extremely valuable aid for growing—soot. It has a simple function: to darken the surface of the soil so that in the cold weather more of the sun's heat is absorbed and retained. You can do the same thing, I suppose, with black plastic: but the fine black layers of soot are not only pleasanter to the eye but allow air to penetrate the soil. Soot is not a soil food; it is merely a mechanical conditioner, a simple organic substance that prolongs growth.

Straw

You can use straw as an aid to organic growing, and bales of it make excellent building blocks for many purposes. I have seen a vegetable garden raised from the ground and entirely walled by small straw bales, and the drainage was perfect. Although the vegetables had to be watered every day, the aerated soil full of earthworms was a wonderful growing medium. You can build a compost bin whose sides are composed of small bales of straw. As the straw breaks down it can be incorporated into the compost so that you are ensuring a complete absorption of all materials in a highly efficient manner. The initial cost of the straw bales is more than balanced by the increased productivity of your garden.

Leaf Mould

Organic growing is the process of using, or re-using, materials that would otherwise be classed as waste. Intelligently applied, they can contribute most of the needs of the next growing cycle. Leaves, instead of burning their way out of this world in a spiral of blue smoke, can be pressed into service again on earth, literally *pressed*. Make a simple wire cage from scrap timber and chicken wire 90 centimetres (3 feet) square and 60 centimetres (2 feet) deep and tip the leaves into this container as they are raked up; then press them down very tightly. This compressing of the leaves (quite different from composting methods) excludes air—for our aim is to produce pure leaf mould, and this is how it is made. On forested hillsides you have all seen pockets of leaf mould at the base of trees, usually on the high side of the trees where leaves washed down by heavy rains have caught against the tree-stump. This crumbly, blackish-brown spongy material often has shed bark mixed with it, forming a leaf and bark mould that is stronger than leaf mould on its own. The leaves from deciduous trees such as oak and beech and birch and larch and ash, those from deciduous fruit-trees such as peaches, plums and cherries, and those from eucalypts, are naturally different in composition; and you may like to make a pot-pourri mixture—remembering that the gumleaves will take longer to break down than the rest. Here you have pure mineral content, without the potash but with trace minerals in abundance; the trees' deep roots have drawn this sustenance up into the leaves and flowers and fruit. You can join in this recycling, returning the compressed leaves into the top layer of soil. And several hundred or several thousand years from now the heavy minerals will once again have filtered down and down through soil layers for the tree-roots to dredge them up again.

Leaf mould is often highly acid. It is eminently suitable for growing ferns and begonias and most indoor plants, and can be used for potting orchids and native plants. A wander round a piece of waste land with an empty bucket can be both interesting and profitable, and you'll usually come home with a bucketful of leaf mould. It is found in the most unlikely places: in scrubby bush, washed into crevices between stones, against tree boles, backed into creek corners. Usually it's under a top layer of twigs and bark and refuse that, if left there, would be broken down in several years into the same stuff. Scoop away this twiggy overlay and fill your bucket with the rich, brownish spongy mould. This type of compost is especially suitable for maidenhair ferns and for any plants that grow in semi-shade, such as azaleas, camellias and rhododendrons.

Don't forget to stamp those leaves down hard in any enclosure where you put them: unlike compost, they must be without air. A thick, compacted layer of them should take from three to four years to break down completely into the true mouldy condition. This may seem a long while to wait for returns, but once you've waited you will, of course, have

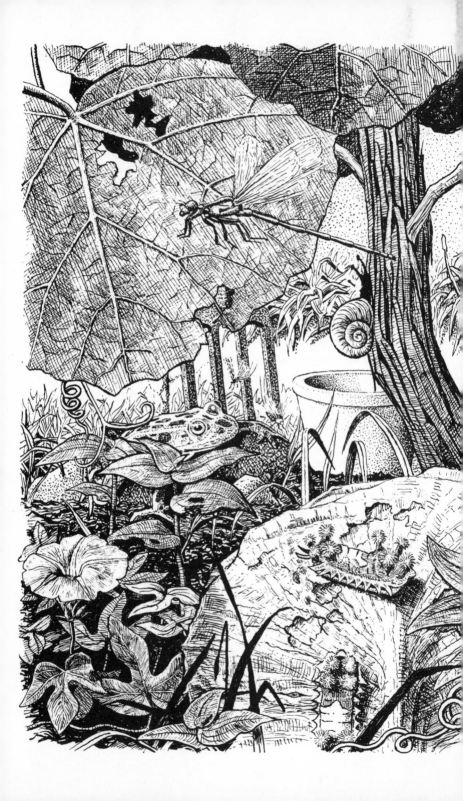

leaf material each year as you go along. Do not put in any leaves of the resinous trees such as camphor laurel or pittosporum, or pine or conifer branches, for these all contain compounds that inhibit moulds and preserve vegetation rather than let it break down at normal speed.

Whatever you do, don't add lantana to leaf mould: this plant is, to my mind, one of the only rogues that I know of—a true scoundrel in the vegetable world who should be eradicated for the good of the rest of the tribe. The tamed garden varieties of lantana are different altogether from the pink-and-yellow-flowered menace that goes berserk. It can poison the soil, and its leaves dropping beside other plants add toxic resinous substances that last for years.

Seaweed

Seaweed is a vegetable, but it has few things in common with its above-ground relatives. Staying in the one spot in the ocean and reproducing itself, it has a totally different way of assimilating its food. It has no flowers or seeds, and it attaches itself by anchors or holdfasts to rock faces or the sea-floor. It does not have sap to rise or fall, and every cell all over its body absorbs food and manufactures life energy. This is why it is so valuable in our gardens.

The heavier minerals and all the good plant food washed away down our concrete gutters and hosed off our driveways and processed through our sewerage systems eventually finds its way down to the sea. Everything that is denuded from the land in the way of good (and, unfortunately, bad) material winds up in the ocean. Seaweeds can start here another complete recycling: they absorb only the good and necessary things for animal and plant life and totally ignore the chemicals and synthetics and artificially constructed compounds floating past them in residual wastes. Seaweed *can* be killed off in creeks and estuaries if the waste content of the water is excessive, but in the open ocean this does not occur.

Seaweed grows at such a rapid rate that it can supply

abundant food for every backyard gardener, and for his family and his animals, without making even the slightest impression on the vast reserves still hidden beneath the blue waters. Seaweed, and kelp in particular—and dulse, too, its close relative—contains almost every known mineral necessary for human and plant life. The trace minerals that became recognised several generations ago as necessary for our depleted pastures and gardens are found naturally in kelp. You don't need to buy all those fancy pink pellets to give your garden zip and zing: just take a trip to the seaside, if you can. On the sea coast there are masses of seaweed at high-tide mark, and after a storm you will find so much of it that you could load up a truckful and still hardly make any impression. I have what I call my survival kit in my motor-car, consisting of a fork, secateurs, a pair of thick gloves, and plastic bags (the large size for seaweed collecting). I have a favourite area on the mid and lower North Coast of New South Wales, where the rocky continental shelf precipitates masses of seaweed on the beach after a south-easterly blow, and I pick strands of kelp and load them into the plastic bags. The slimy, slithery strands can be placed directly on the garden beds (on the rose-bushes, on the vegetables and the annuals and the shrubs); or they can be added to the compost bins. Sometimes I spread them out on a flat rock to dry for a day or two before handling them at all; but don't leave them any longer, because seaweed exposed in hot sun decomposes too rapidly, losing many of its organic properties. If you put it on the surface of your garden beds, just chop it lightly in with a hoe, or fork it in a little so that it can decompose there to some purpose in feeding the plants around it.

You may wonder what happens to the salt in seaweed. Well, it's a strange thing, seaweed does not absorb sodium chloride. It absorbs sodium ions and chloride ions and this type of sodium and chlorine does not worry your plants or your animals or yourself at all. In fact, North Atlantic farmers have been cropping vegetables for hundreds of years with seaweed washed right up over their fields in heavy storms. What better work-free, trouble-free, natural way to replace trace and heavy minerals than to let the sea expend the effort for you!

Adding seaweed to your compost enables it to break down into the most complete plant food you could ever need or design in the laboratory. I am not going to tell you exact scientific quantities because Nature does not work that way and neither do I. It is a commonsense thing: some kelp in the compost is fine, but a bin composed entirely of seaweed is not. A little of everything and a state of balance is achieved.

If you live away from the seaside and cannot get fresh kelp you can buy granulated kelp from your health store and sprinkle this into compost. You can also use the store-bought kelp for house plants as a complete fertiliser. Use only a little at first until you work out your plants' needs, sprinkling it over the surface of the soil and turning it lightly in, then following it through with a good soaking for the pots. House plants grow much better, though, if the entire potting medium consists of the blackish warm contents of your compost bin to which kelp has been added during its making. You can also buy liquid seaweed mixtures that are ideal for gardeners who have little time and little inclination to mess about with composting. The liquid mixtures can be used as a complete fertiliser for every plant that grows. Fish-meal fertiliser is a good liquid manure too, with every needed plant nutrient in it.

Bull-kelp, the brownish-green seaweed with the thick strappy leaves, seems to be the best for gardens, but you can also use many of the other varieties with varying degrees of benefit. All kelp is good kelp. Make it a regular part of your week-end outings to the beach to gather any that's lying about; but remember that the best results come from kelp that has been washed up in the last twenty-four hours or so, rather than from kelp that has been lying farther up the beach for many days or weeks.

The only place you can do without seaweed is in a fresh-water aquarium! You can even bath in seaweed, and as well as feeling somewhat like a mermaid or merman you can be sure it is doing your skin a power of good with the soft natural mucilage it contains tightening and firming tissues all over your body. Seaweed face-packs as a regular beauty treatment can do all sorts of things to rejuvenate skins lacking in those minute but essential trace elements we have trouble finding from other sources. You don't really know whether your skin needs boron or molybdenum or cobalt, but the general effect after giving it a seaweed face-pack is that it must have needed *something*—and the seaweed supplied it.

Dogs and cats can have seaweed granules sprinkled over their meals. My dog nearly eats her way through the bottom of her food dish to get every last flake of greyish-green kelp from the bowl. Her bounding good health and energy, the silkiness and general texture of her coat and the clearness of her eye, show what kelp and natural foods can do for an eight-year-old dog.

PESTS AND DISEASES

Pests and diseases are the serpents in the organic grower's Eden. When you first make the vow to change your gardening habits, when you throw away your plastic packets, and your bottles of evil-smelling chemicals marked 'Poison', you may wonder what is going to help you when the roses become covered with aphis, the lemon-tree with its yellow-green new leaves has blackish-winged visitors curling up the shoots, or your vegetable patch has the white cabbage moth hovering around it. You may also wonder what to do when the chrysanthemums suffer from eelworm in the soil and clubroot strikes the potatoes. 'This idyllic method sounds marvellous,' you may say. 'But what happens when pests of all descriptions come to live on my beautiful healthy plants?' One answer, which you may not easily believe during the first season or two, is that insect pests attack organically grown plants less and less. But what natural methods of controlling insect or disease invasion are you to use during the first few seasons? Nature, as usual, is ten steps in front and has shown us all sorts of natural ways of deterring insects and soil pests and diseases.

Let's start with the simplest ways. I have a picture in my mind of my grandmother marching around her vegetable patch at night with a torch and a little box of salt, 'doing the snails'. It sounds a little fiendish; but something has to be done to head the snails off, and a quick method is just to drop a pinch of salt on any snail or slug that is doing a re-connaissance round the carrot seedlings or pansies. Osmotic pressure does the rest: all the fluids in the unfortunate animal bubble out, and it dehydrates rapidly and dies. Complete the cycle of Nature and return the dried-up shell-covered bodies to the compost bin the next morning. Even dead snails have a contribution to make to natural growing.

There is another way: Natural barriers can be set up between the prized plants and the marauding snails and slugs. A snail's existence depends on being able to get back into its shell after feeding at night, and if you can prevent this you will either kill off the snail or it will realise that the barrier you have erected is insurmountable and dangerous for snails. Sprinkle coarse sawdust right round your vegetable patch or round any area you wish to keep snail-free. This band of sawdust should be about an inch (2 centimetres) in height, and the coarser it is the better. The particles of dust and coarser wood slivers stick to the snail and prevent its getting back into its shell. Some snails are sensible, and spend the entire night circling round the barrier, trying to find a way in; others stupidly try to crash the barrier, and perish miserably soon after.

On a mid-evening snail hunt you will discover all sorts of night-life about in your garden. There will be moths and tiny flying ants, perhaps, and crickets on the move, and if you are lucky and have natural water or seepage near by you may get a frog or two with its headlights shining in the beam from your torch. I have three different varieties of frog in and around my garden where the natural watercourse of an old creek is always slightly damp and the frogs dearly love to sit with their backs under moist rocks and stones. Leave any frogs in peace in your garden, for they will eat all sorts of insect larvae and predators and their chorus in wet weather can be most relaxing. You can leave the garden lizards running about, too, because they eat all sorts of minute insect eggs, and their burrowing under fallen leaves keeps air circulating and prevents fungous diseases from breeding.

Large insects that sit in one spot on fruit-tree or plant are no problem. Walking quietly along the rows of herbs or vegetables or amongst the succulent-leaved annuals, you can spot the grasshoppers or stink-bugs or other sitting insects and easily collect them. If you have qualms about killing animals, remember that those little bodies will be providing more natural animal content for the compost heap. When you lay the dead insects on Nature's funeral pyre, you may be sending them out of this world to come back again in the molecules of a naturally fed iris blossom or ripe red apple.

There are two major classes of insect pests, the leaf-chewers and the sap-suckers. Leaf-chewers are often large insects such as grasshoppers and beetles and bugs, and if you do not wish to spend the time hunting them individually you can make up a simple spray mixture that is not only lethal but breaks up in the soil, leaving not a trace of inorganic pollutant. There are sprays for sucking insects, too, but I prefer to mix all my sprays in one bucket so that I get a broad-spectrum cover of suckers, chewers, biters and crawlers. To a basic nicotine spray I add garlic corms and rosemary and lavender if my bushes are big enough to rob; and sometimes I add rhubarb leaves and even one of my favourite fungicide herbs, *Equisetum arvense* or horsetail. If you are interested in making up quantities of organic sprays, a good

little booklet is *Pest Control without Poisons*. It is published
by the Henry Doubleday Research Association, of Bocking,
Braintree, in Essex, England, and contains a wealth of
technical information as to quantities and measurements.
But here is a very simple recipe for an effective spray: take a
foul-smelling mound of cigarette butts (saved for you by
unregenerate friends) and use these as the basis of the spray
mixture; or buy a pipe-type tobacco. If these butts have a
filter tip, weigh about 113 grams; if they are plain or roll-
your-own type, about 56 grams. What you want is a net
quantity of about 56 grams of tobacco. Add these smelly
ends (or the bought tobacco) to about 4 litres of water—
perhaps a little more, for some of the water will boil away—
and to this mixture add several other ingredients to give a
complete cover for any insects you have not been able to
catch, head off, or persuade to move elsewhere.

The first additive is garlic, for this quantity four good-size
cloves. (The clove is the individual segment of which garlic
corms are composed.) Then add a good handful of well-
chopped rosemary or well-chopped lavender, including the
stems of each, sliced with kitchen scissors or cut on the
chopping board, and bruised and crushed so that their oil
content goes into the boiling water. To this solution you can
add, either half-way through the boiling or at the end of it,
about half a cake of pure yellow soap which has been soaked
the previous night in water, softening it so that it will dissolve
easily. Keep one particular large boiling vessel for this spray-
making, and paint SPRAY—POISON on the side of it so that
every member of the family knows it is something *not* to
cook the Christmas ham in! Boil this quite startlingly indi-
vidual-smelling mixture for approximately one half-hour. If
the family complains, you can boil it out in the open air on
a camp stove; and if you do boil it up in a house where there
are still cigarette-smokers, it will go a long way towards
convincing them of the poisonous nature of the stuff they are
putting into their lungs.

This is a basic mixture to deal with animal predators, but if you suspect or know there may be fungous spores about, such as those of black spot and mildew, you can add to your spray some horsetail, *Equisetum arvense*, which may be a little harder for you to obtain from gardening sources but is available through your health store in the form of equisitum tea. Add to the spray mixture, in the last few minutes of its boiling time, a good handful of the dried equisetum herb, roughly 56 grams; as the mixture cools, the high silica content will be drawn from the herb.

When the mixture has cooled—and you can leave it overnight with all the herb material still in it—strain it through fine muslin or a piece of nylon. Then store the brown evil-smelling liquid in a glass or plastic container with an airtight lid. I use 2-litre wine flagons, preferring glass to plastic which tends to absorb. Lastly, and importantly label the container clearly POISON, put it on a high shelf in your laundry or garden shed, and make sure it is kept away from children, pets, and non-gardeners. It is certainly highly toxic, and must not accidentally fall into the wrong hands. Use the spray within the next two weeks: it goes mouldy if kept longer.

For spraying, mix one part of this mixture with four parts of water. The 4 litres of concentrate will give you rather more than 20 litres of spray, sufficient to cover a good-sized home garden. Spraying should not need to be done more than once every two weeks, even in the months of the year when plants are most susceptible to insect or fungus invasion; and don't spray at all unless you see signs of damage. There is no need whatsoever to give a healthy plant a dose of poison, no matter how safely degradable that poison becomes: the less spray the better, always. Any vegetables or edible plants are ready for you to take to the table two weeks after spray has been applied. Do not eat any of them before this time, for though the spray mixture is totally organic and will break down in the soil completely, leaving no harmful effects, eating vegetables or fruit sprayed with it before that two weeks has elapsed could make you feel a little queasy. You can apply this spray through a watering-can over foliage and soil, but this can be wasteful, and a garden spray is better. Adjust the spray nozzle to a wide spread and work your way up and down the vegetable rows or over the fruit-trees. Don't forget to spray under leaves, too, for most of the spores of fungous diseases work their way up the plant from the soil, and many are splashed up there by raindrops bouncing them against the underside of low leaves.

The more efficiently and intelligently you garden organically the less insect and fungus problem you will have. Spraying your garden every two weeks is necessary only when insects are troublesome or humid conditions have brought harmful fungus invasion; and this period has been nominated because it is the length of time during which the spray gives protection. Of course, if it rains immediately after you have applied the spray, you have lost a lot of it and may have to re-spray sooner. Prevention is more admirable (and easier) than cure; but even natural, organically simple sprays like this one should not be put on vegetables and flower gardens unless they are absolutely required.

When you do spray, make sure your entire family knows you have done so, and keep a little chart somewhere in the kitchen or in the tool-shed so that no one will pick vegetables or fruit for the table without consulting the chart to see when the last spraying was done.

If you prefer a powder-type insect repellent, you can use pure pyrethrum, which is the white flower of *Chrysanthemum cinerariifolium*, the South African pyrethrum daisy, not to be confused with the garden pyrethrum, which is of no value at all in combating pests. If you can buy this pyrethrum dust pure or mixed only with organic substances like derris dust, this is fine for your garden; but in many countries it is not obligatory for pesticide manufacturers to list on their labels all the ingredients that are present. You may see on the nurseryman's shelves rows and rows of pesticide or fungicide products that contain either pyrethrum or derris or both; but, if you can, ring the supplier to ask him whether the preparation contains only these substances or whether there are other inorganic preparations mixed with them. If you can get either of these dusts or both of them in a pure state they are an excellent insect-deterring combination. Apply these in the same circumstances—only when insects are about—and do not eat the vegetable or fruit until approximately two weeks have elapsed.

One very good reason for never using synthetic (non-organic) sprays is that they can kill not only the predator insects and the harmful fungus but everything else, including earthworms and bees. You know now how valuable the earthworm is to the health of your garden; and the work done for you by the bee population is just as important in pollinating and fertilising to give heavy crops in orchards and vegetable gardens. You would not want to have to get up at five o'clock in the morning to spend an hour or two running around your pumpkin vines and your apple-trees and your strawberry patch with a feather, going from one flower to the next to make sure that pollen is transferred: and this is what you would have to do if the bees in your garden did not do it for you. Any spray or dust used to control insects should be applied late in the evening after the bees have gone to bed: to catch all the other day-feeders, and some of the early night-feeders too, without stunning all the bees when they should be busily carrying pollen. A direct application of the nicotine spray to a bee can most certainly kill it; and even an odd splash or two in passing can stun it badly. Do your spraying at dusk, not first thing in the morning.

If your garden is badly affected by black spot or mildew after humid weather, an excellent old-fashioned remedy is the famous Bordeaux Mixture. It is still as good at deterring fungus as it ever was, and it is another spray that breaks down completely after a couple of weeks. Buy 170 grams (6 ounces) of copper sulphate or bluestone and dissolve this (in that same vessel marked SPRAY—POISON) in 2 litres (3 pints) of boiling water. Stand this aside, and in a separate vessel (preferably one you can throw away afterwards) put 140 grams (5 ounces) of lime. Add enough water to this to make 2 litres (3 pints); then add 140 grams (5 ounces) of treacle to the limewater in the container and boil the lime and treacle mixture for about fifteen minutes, stirring it occasionally. Let this lime/treacle mixture cool, then add it to the bluestone mixture, which has also cooled. If there is any sediment in the lime mixture, strain it before mixing with the other. Add enough water to make the mixture up to 18 litres (4 gallons). I have found that the best container for this spray is a plastic 18-litre (4-gallon) can, since it is difficult to get a glass vessel that will hold so much. The mixture is corrosive to metals, and should not be stored in tins or any other metal container. The mixture, sealed from the air, should keep for many weeks. If you want this spray to adhere to plant foliage rather than soil, don't skimp on the treacle. If the mixture tends to set during storage, stand the container in hot sunlight or running hot water before using.

There is a natural type spray you can use for weeds, but it may also kill your precious plants. It is better used for areas where you wish to remove all vegetation, and I use it on my stubborn patches of wandering jew or oxalis when there are no other plants I value near by. One corner of my garden is particularly hard to weed by hand because big boulders and natural shelves of rock make it difficult to get at; and since there is nothing in this area except tree and shrub specimens I save my aching back by spraying instead of grubbing out the invaders. This spray is simple and works effectively on a purely mechanical level by excluding air from the leaves so that they cannot transpire, and they die. It is made from ordinary household kerosene to which has been added a dissolved half-cake of yellow washing soap. You spray this undiluted if the weeds are thickly matted, or it can be broken down and emulsified slightly with about an equal quantity of water. This breaking down must be done with extreme care, for it is necessary to heat the kerosene and water together with the soap, and you can imagine what would happen if such a mixture boiled over! Whatever you do, make up this type of spray outside, in an open area away from shrubs and trees and fences, so that if any unlooked-for accident occurs you won't set the house—or yourself—on fire. I really prefer to use just that little bit more kerosene (it's very cheap) and play safe rather than brew up such a potentially lethal mixture over heat. Kerosene can be used along pathway edges or stone flagging or driveways to deter weeds from germinating at all. It will break down into natural harmless residues, and it has the effect of inhibiting growth, sometimes for months.

With these three simple, basic sprays you can control unwanted visitors, either animal or vegetable, bearing in mind that the less you use them the better. Obviously spraying should be done on a day with a minimum of wind so that it will not spread where you don't want it to: spray at dusk when the wind has usually dropped.

GREEN MANURING

Green manuring is a valuable form of soil improvement; it not only fertilises but controls small harmful bacteria. The best crops for green manuring are those of the legume family, such as peas and clovers and lupins. These can be planted not only on an agricultural scale to improve soil, but in your own backyard to sweeten soil and add to its nitrogen content. I had an area of poor bush soil that was sandy and pale; so I planted seeds of lupins over it; and when the plants appeared and grew they provided a cover for the soil so that the moisture content increased and (I knew) the nitrogen content, too. Many legumes are better if dug in at peak budding and first flowering time, but lupins contain more nitrogen at a later stage; and I prefer to dig in at this later stage because it always seems such a pity to turn the crop under at the peak of its beauty. With lupins, you get the benefit both ways: pleasure to look upon, and a soil conditioning when they begin literally to run to seed. The yellow lupins are excellent for this, as are the single blue ones; but don't use the enormous garden hybrids bred for display, because much of their work energy is channelled into oversize flowers. After this first manuring with lupin plants, well chopped up and spaded in, I planted yet another setting of seed of the same variety, and this time I interspersed the plantings with small herbs from my previous garden. Some of these treasures were only a few centimetres in height, and the terraces into which they were transplanted were sunny and scorching even in early autumn; so I gave the new plants a lupin squad to protect them. The health and vigour of these herbs was amazing, by the time the lupins were ready to turn in as green manure. I chopped the lupins all in, with their tiny immature seed-pods, turning them lightly under the top 6 inches (15 centimetres) or so of soil. At the ready, in my compost bin, was a load of black rich food that I spaded on top of the turned-under lupins and up against the stems of the vigorously growing herbs. These terraces of herbs are a prime example of healthy plants in healthy soil.

Mustard, as a green manure crop, seems to work as stinging nettles do, giving the soil not only green growing matter to provide humus as it breaks down but vegetable iron that stirs nearby plants into vigorous growth. As the mustard plants grow, use the leaves in your salad bowl, or cooked as a vegetable—and what a wealth of minerals and trace minerals these leaves contain! Their iron and calcium riches are just as good for humans as they are for soil. Mustard grows very fast: it can be sown in vegetable beds before you sow the seeds or seedlings of the vegetables and dug in soon after the plants appear. The common pea plants grow quickly, too; and they

germinate well, are cheap to buy, and have the same nitrogenous soil-building value. So put in a clump or two of these if you
can bear to dig them in before the pale young seed-pods begin
to form, depriving yourself of the joy of tasting immature
peas steamed in their pods.

If you are growing peas for their own sake, eat them when
they are fully formed as pods but before the peas inside have
rounded and taken shape. Then you can whip off the woody
ends and use them swizzled around in a little oil, with diced
capsicum and onion and celery stems, for an excellent source
of vitamin C and a new taste sensation. The true Chinese
delicacies used for this dish are the variety of sugar peas
known as snow peas, but you can do a similar job with tender,
immature garden peas grown naturally.

COMPANION PLANTING

The object of companion planting is to make it unneccssary
to interfere at all with plants that supply one another's needs.
Like humans, plants are individuals with different requirements for their health and happiness. And if one plant's
excreta can provide the next plant's food without our meddling, if one plant thrives in the company of another, by all
means let them live as Nature intended. By carefully obser-
ving which plants grow well together, build up your own
collection of companion-plant information. There is a very
useful book by Helen Philbrick and Richard P. Gregg called
Companion Plants (Stuart and Watkins, London, 1967) that
tells you, without giving reasons, which plants like to be
with other plants. The information may not always apply
to the climate or soil in your garden, and you must supplement and qualify it from your own observation and experience. *Look* at where your plants are growing; have a look at
a patch of bushland; and observe whether one plant next
to another seems to thrive in its company. Nature excels in
compatibility placement, and her patches of weeds are living

textbooks on how to cultivate crops by choosing plants that get along with each other on a give-and-take basis. Using such knowledge domestically, we find, for instance, that borage helps strawberries to fruit more abundantly, while strawberries add to the health and disease-resistance of borage plants; horseradish plants at the end of potato rows inhibit many of the soil pests and diseases affecting potatoes, because of the 'antibiotic' action of horseradish roots in the soil. It is said that basil will not grow beside rue and that rue will not grow under fig-trees; but I have for many years planted rue and basil together to test this theory, and then planted them separately under identical growing conditions, and I have seen no sign of their hating each other in any way.

Much of the companion-plant lore that applies in the Northern Hemisphere in a temperate zone does not apply in the tropics or in Southern continents. This may be because of different magnetic conditions, different vibrations, different composition of soils, different native-type vegetation. So remember this in referring to books on companion planting. My failure to grow sage plants, no matter under what conditions they have been raised or in what growing medium they have been placed, may be an example of vibrationary patterns affecting plants—just as instinctive dislikes occur between human beings. Strangely there is a certain *type* of person who cannot grow parsley, no matter how green their fingers with other plants. Collecting a list of the people I know who have this in common, I find they are all the same kind of person, with a particular biochemical/emotional pattern that apparently parsley does not like. I believe there can be definite plant/human relationships; and apart from soil chemistry and plant anatomy there is more to companion planting than meets the practical eye.

Nature's landscaping consists of tall vegetation where the plants in front need shelter to grow. Plants grow more closely together where there is abundant composting material over their roots, as in forests; and plants grow sparsely on areas of plain where they must compete for the nutriment available. When you place one plant next to another in your garden or orchard or grazing property, consider how you can best use the natural companions available to ensure that the least possible amount of work has to be done to keep your plants healthy. I am not a gardener dedicated to weeding and hoeing and chopping and cutting back and planting out. I like to have time to contemplate and look and learn; and, while sitting and looking at good and bad results, to ask myself 'Why?'

Why has one row of vegetables grown taller than the two rows next to it, or why has a tree died, or why has a shrub grown in the one spot year after year without ever setting a flower? A little common sense can .often show you where *not* to put plants, or how to grow one with another for the maximum benefit of both. For instance, tree-ferns, natives in many parts of the world, grow naturally in gullies and cooler spots and they love compost round their roots, compost that is acid. It would be silly to plant them in a district with a naturally alkaline soil unless you take the trouble to create an acid-soil area that suits them.

The compatibility of strawberries and borage could be of commercial value if it were generally known, for example. And I grow stinging nettles among my herbs and perfumed flowers, because I know this increases their oil content and flavour and perfume, as well as the life and vigour of the hair-roots at the surface. In experimenting in companion planting, you will find that totally dissimilar plants, such as chives and apple-trees, or chives and roses, are very good mates. The soil-sterilising properties of chives protect the apple-tree from scab disease, and the roses from aphis attack. In reverse, the companion-planting technique can eliminate a troublesome weed or a plant you do not care for. Tomatoes planted thickly in an area where you are having trouble with couch-grass runners eliminate this grass, which, though tamed in lawns, can go quite berserk if it gets away from you.

Every organic grower knows that once in a while his garden should be planted with marigolds, which can do a thorough job of cleansing the soil from nematode and eelworm pests. These are *Tagetes*, the African marigold, and it is better to get the plain, common, orange ones rather than the hybridised, overbred, enormous garden varieties. While blazing away in full splendour when other annuals are scarce, they are doing a splendid job for you underground. If you are a chrysanthemum-grower, make it a rule to plant marigolds either beside the chrysanthemums or alternating with each plant in the bed, for chrysanthemums are very susceptible to eelworm attack, and you can lose prize specimens in no time if this pest is not checked.

Study the likes and dislikes of plants in order to learn what they need for maximum growth and health. If you really look at a shrub, an annual, or a vegetable, some of its characteristics should strike you straight away. Is it a plant whose glory is in the leaf growth; is it a plant that has nondescript foliage for twelve months then bursts into showy blossom for two or three weeks; is it a plant that concentrates all its energy in one overgrown flower-bud (as the cabbage does); or is it a plant that must wait to flower or to fruit until conditions are exactly right (as the cactus family does)? If you can, grow one plant with an exaggerated characteristic in one direction next to another plant that has an opposite characteristic, so preserving some sort of balance. Sometimes Nature does this herself; sometimes you can help her. Experiment yourself with these opposites, and with the likes and dislikes of plants one for the other, and you are bound to come up with unusual information. Companion planting is a comparatively recent reintroduction of a very ancient principle, and much remains to be rediscovered about it.

Crop rotation must be practised commercially so that the soil does not become one-sidedly depleted from the growth of only a single type of vegetable or flower. A leaf crop is followed by a flower crop, then a root crop. In your garden, without being obliged to wait a whole season, you can plant a row of one, then a row of another, then a third row, all in the same bed, and do your crop-rotating simultaneously. The root crop takes what roots need and returns to the soil what flowers and fruit perhaps need, so that each row planted side by side keeps that cycle of elements moving through the soil in a living river of foodstuffs available to all the plants at the same time.

Vegetables are traditionally planted in rows—a troop of cabbages, a platoon of carrots, a neat section of rhubarb. Most gardeners believe that vegetables have individual needs and that such a plan makes life easier. If you are not growing commercially, I don't agree. So many vegetables are decorative plants that I often plant a group amongst my flower beds—and not only the decorative ones, either: for some vegetable crops enhance some flower crops, and vice versa. At the moment some winter dwarf peas are flowering, climbing up dead lemon-tree twigs, and I shall soon have the sweet young immature pods to eat raw or chop in with hot vegetable dishes at the last minute before taking them to the table. This bed will then be planted with annuals for a springtime show of leaf and flower; and in the meantime three clumps of arum lilies, wandered in from some other part of the garden, are growing in splendiferous health amongst the pea vines. It may look a little haphazard now, but those spring annuals will have a background companion in the lily family to their mutual benefit. The peas are returning nitrogen to the soil at a great rate, so that garden bed will be in great shape for early annual planting. I have a magnificent plant of rhubarb in the corner of two vegetable beds, and I intend to arrange a few more clumps at suitable corners where they can give shade to more tender vegetables near them. My vegetable garden is 'landscaped', too—no rows or lines, just happy groups of dissimilar plants chatting to each other and taking out of the soil and putting back in for their neighbours. There are odd clumps of chives amongst the vegetable chicory, keeping unwanted insects away and contributing organic sulphur to the soil for the cabbages and chicory. And there is a little bush of marjoram next to where my tomatoes will grow in the warmer weather. The marjoram will condition the soil so that tomato bugs will not like the taste of the ripening plant and will not be a pest. The tomatoes will have the fine spicy flavour of just a touch of marjoram. There are clumps of wild garlic here and there amongst the vegetables, and some Welsh onions, which flourish right through the winter months when the other members of the onion family are dormant underground. Any planting of onions helps other vegetables, and most vegetables benefit from a light flavour of onion coming through. Onion family members do a tremendous job in the soil in an antibiotic fashion, deterring harmful soil bacteria and encouraging the beneficial strains.

Watercress

Watercress is one of those virtuous vegetables with so many minerals and vitamins that it's a shame not to have it growing where you can pick it yourself. Its natural companion is pure running water, and you are unlikely to have a clear running stream in your garden. But, using simple materials, you can provide the true companion needed by watercress. First dig a hole about 45 centimetres deep and 90 centimetres in diameter (18 inches by 3 feet), either on the shady side of a tall fence or in shade from a wall of green somewhere in the garden. In the bottom of this hole throw some pieces of old rusty iron or tin cans, and a good shovelful of well-rotted manure or of blood-and-bone. Add some torn-up scraps of old hessian or underfelt or some shovelfuls of peat-moss to give the new watercress plants loose porous material under their roots, so that the moisture you are going to drip onto them will be held for long enough in the hole. Shovel the soil back over this mess in the bottom of the hole until it's within 10 or 12 centimetres (4–5 inches) of the surface. Now sow your watercress seeds here, or if you can get watercress plants from the markets or mountain streams with the roots still attached and not too dried out you can lay these around the edge of the hole with the roots towards the centre of it. Leave a shallowish depression towards the centre, so that even if you are sowing seeds here you can ensure that moisture given will be retained long enough. Cover the roots with a piece of old hessian or sacking and fill up the hole on top of this with more soil to about 5 or 6 centimetres (2–3 inches) in depth. This should leave you with a shallow depression sloping towards the centre. Over this depression you can put up what looks like an Indian tepee support: three posts or stakes of some description, either wooden or metal, arranged in a triangle with the top ends wired and bound strongly together and the bottoms pushed firmly and deeply into the ground around the hole. Suspend under this tripod a large container of water, with a hole pierced in the bottom of it, a hole that will allow the water to drip onto the plants at the rate of no more than 9 litres (2 gallons) every twelve hours. Experiment with the container and its rate of flow first, starting with a tiny hole, before you plant the watercress. You will soon find how big the hole has to be to provide a constant drip, drip, drip of water. This arrangement can look quite neat and tidy if you use your imagination with poles and containers, and it can be set in a part of the garden that is not your showpiece and is handy to the water supply. This may sound like a lot of trouble, but the concentrated food value of watercress makes it worth trying. When you are cutting it for the table, make sure you cut only the green tips above the hessian, leaving the roots below in the water-saturated ground. Without its companion of water, this valuable plant would not be able to grow at all. The water carries the iron from those rusty cans and waste lumps of metal to the watercress roots, which absorb free ions from the mineral and pass it on to us in a potent form of vegetable iron.

WATER

Pure water is rare in our modern world—and distilled water has not the type of purity I mean.

The purest natural water I have found myself was in creeks and streams close to the peak of Mount Kosciusko. Here, on these ancient mountains, I found water such as I had never tasted in my life before, run-off water from melted snow that had fallen on the peaks of the Snowy Mountains six to ten months before and had been purified by its action of running over glacial-era granite and sedges and mosses and alpine herbage. It appeared to me to have collected ambrosia—or such was the taste of the natural elements acquired in its passage from the very crown of the mountain peaks washed clean by melting snow. This water tasted as all water should taste, alive and pure, and with a distinctive flavour of its own that you might call 'liquid Nature'. In our towns and cities we drink a pale imitation of what real water can be.

If you wish to taste the true flavour of water as it should be, sprout wheatgrass and cut off the green growing tips of the shoots to add to a container of water. After about twelve to twenty hours, remove the shoots, and the water tastes as you never remember water tasting before. It has become biochemically free from many of the substances that civilisation has added to it.

Every living organism must have water, or the moisture in the air from water vapour. Without moisture in the cells of the body, men and animals and plants dehydrate and die. It is obviously so with plants, and even the plants that grow on the stoniest and most arid of all deserts could not survive without some source of moisture. The cactus stores its own; the date palms dredge up moisture from oases deep under desert sands; plants in the lush jungles of tropical areas transpire water through their leaves, making prolific growth.

It is only by means of water that plants can use the minerals and the enzyme substances and the microscopic material present in soils. Water is the carrier, taking these substances from one plant to another through the soil, from above the ground to below it, from below the ground through the roots of plants to their growing stems and leaves. Every cell of every living thing needs water.

Although no plant can survive without water, you can kill a plant more easily by over-watering it than by giving it only a meagre ration. Over-watering of plants in a temperate climate makes them behave like tropical plants whose sur-face-rooting systems have abundant moisture presented to them at ground level, so that they have little need to dive down searching for it. This is fine as long as the moisture is kept up to them; but the minute you stop watering, or if there is a long dry spell, or if your garden does not have suf-ficient mulch and compost on top of the soil, the surface roots facing happily upwards waiting for their next drink will be scorched and the plant will die. In organic growing the precious water is retained underground and not wasted in evaporation.

Today in my garden I lifted up a layer of compost on top of a new terrace bed where I have planted several shrubs and where the hot afternoon sun has beaten down for about ten days. I had not watered this bed. Below the 7-centimetre (5-inch) layer of compost mulch the soil was damp and loose and easily moved about with one finger, so that I could open up the soil surface easily below. The terrace bed below this, which had purposely not been mulched at all and had similar shrubs planted in it, I had had to water three times within that same period. The soil surface was compacted hard and tight like concrete. By composting well, you can save all those trips out to change the hose, and you can cut your watering by at least one-third over dry periods. Plant roots grow towards moisture, and you have little need to coddle the deep-rooting shrubs and trees after the initial growth and bedding-in stages, for they will dive right down to deeper levels where the water is retained. It is only surface-rooting annuals and some vegetables that must be kept supplied with water at surface level; and composting techniques can strengthen the surface root system so that even when water is not in good supply the plant's roots are well protected and may dive deeper looking for it.

The consistency of the top 10 to 15 centimetres (4 to 6 inches) of soil should be like that of a damp sponge; and so it will be if you have a good layer of mulch on the surface. If the soil texture is heavy and clayey it will need humus and organic material (such as peat-moss and plenty of dolomite) to loosen it so that there will be drainage away from the roots of the plant. Apart from true aquatic plants, which must have their roots in water, all plants need their roots to be damp but not soggy. Water that does not drain away is deadly; too much water on sandy soils, where the particle size is smaller and moisture will drain away quickly, is not so dangerous. Terracing of garden beds aids in the retention of water mechanically: whatever run-off there is will be gradual rather than cataract-like, and periods of heavy rain will not be damaging because the rain-water can run down terraces and pass other plant roots as it goes in a slower, more sedate fashion. Water that is *running* is what plants need rather than water that is stationary. You know how your house-plants react if you over-water them, and the saucer underneath fills up, and they sit for a week, maybe longer, with cold, wet feet. Some of the more delicate varieties can be dead before you have a chance to find out why. Running water leaves natural channels for waste products to escape; brackish or still water gives a fighting chance to all the wrong kind of bacteria, which may prolong their stay instead of being moved on.

It is better to give plants a good soaking at longer intervals rather than short, ineffective sprinkling. Every good gardening book tells you this, and organic gardeners go a step farther, maintaining that with good soil husbandry—mulching and composting, following natural procedures—water or the lack of it can be made less damaging. *Use* the properties of water to spread plant nutrients about your garden. Use it in contour terracing so that every drop is put to work. Use it intelligently so that the food the plants need is carried by it with the least possible interference from you.

CHANGING OVER TO ORGANIC GARDENING METHODS

If you've now decided to banish all synthetic sprays and fertilisers and trace elements and to start anew with organic gardening, how do you get rid of the poisonous residues, the harmful inorganic substances built up in your garden over many years?

One way to regain the natural balance of a healthy growing medium in the top of your soil is to use wheatgrass sprouts. Spread on wet earth a thick sprinkling of wheat-seeds, and cover this planting with sheets of plastic or newspapers weighted down at the corners with either stones or pegging stakes, so that as the wheat germinates it will lift the paper or plastic slightly, enabling air to reach the growing sprouts. When the thick stand of wheatgrass is about 7–12 centimetres (3–5 inches) tall turn the entire mat the roots will have formed completely over—just like an upside-down sod of turf—and replace this mat on the soil surface. Make a second sowing of wheat on top of this, and when the sprouts have reached the same height in the same manner you will have a dense blanket of growth on this area of soil. Then lift this double sod and chop it lightly, breaking it up and and incorporating it with the top few centimetres of soil. Repeat this procedure twice more in order to cleanse the topsoil of any residues of artificial substances left over from your unenlightened days. The wheat germinates best in temperate conditions, and in more humid weather you may find it mildews a little; but we are not looking here for an edible product, only a rejuvenation treatment for the topsoil. This process cleanses soil that has been heavily fertilised artificially, so that you can start growing naturally. The wheat-seed should be kept moist but not waterlogged during the sprouting and growing period, and usually sufficient moisture is retained under the plastic or newspaper for this purpose.

While you are waiting for your garden to produce the naturally grown plants, you must be doubly vigilant in your methods of insect and disease control. A human body needs time to adjust when changing from a bad to a better diet; and a garden, too, can experience strange re-balancing and adjustment problems during this change-over period. We learn how a living soil can almost look after itself by watching what happens to it in different patterns of weed growth, of water retention, of insect behaviour when the chemical composition of the soil and the plants changes. Changes occur, too, in the flowering times and fruiting times of many plants. It may take one or two growing seasons before they settle down to enjoy a natural way of living.

Keep up your composting during this interim period, and use the compost as fast as it becomes available. This is what the plants are craving, for physical insulation and protection, and also for their biochemical needs. The wheatgrass treatment is mostly suitable for fallow areas of ground, or for freshly dug plots before replanting. It is not necessary to empty your garden of everything growing in it before changing over to natural methods. Allow the plants growing there to do their share of the work too, exchanging minerals and growth substances through the soil and the air from one to another; and let their roots keep on dredging up for you the good things that have filtered down into the subsoil. A soil containing any vegetation is healthier than a soil stripped of vegetable life, as the farmers of the newly created dustbowls of America discovered too late.

Roses may bloom in winter or spring-fruiting trees may set fruit in autumn for a season or two until the newly restored natural conditions allow the plants to settle into their normal growth pattern. With organic methods, you are assured of the health of your own garden, and you know you are not guilty of draining or blowing or seeping from your property any harmful substances that can affect your neighbours or contribute to the self-inflicted toxicity we have been perpetuating. Remember, never use any methods of insect or disease control unless you absolutely must, and apply these only at the minimal dose. Allow Nature to play her part; for if we humbly and earnestly try to understand her ways of producing equilibrium, we can learn much. She is not called Mother Nature without reason.

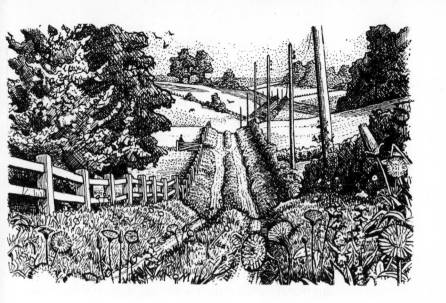

6

Wild Plants and Weeds

A weed is a plant whose usefulness to man has not yet been recognised. You may or may not agree with this definition, and if you're a gardener fighting with oxalis and onionweed and creeping marshmallow you may disagree vigorously. Weeds are the plants that come up when you don't want them to, the plants that thrive when your cabbages don't—so you blame them for the failure or poorness in quality of the plants you want to grow. But malign them as you will, you won't stop them. Weeds spring up out of impossible ground in impossible conditions at an impossible rate of growth. How and why do they keep doing this? Have they some secret that is lost to our daffodils and our poppies and our tomato plants, giving them the vigour to survive?

Weeds can just happen to grow at a particular time in a particular place, then disappear, springing up in patches elsewhere, or dying off altogether, or hibernating for a season or many seasons before suddenly reappearing in the same spot. They are well equipped to face their survival battles, the majority of them having what could be called time-capsule or time-release seeds that vary tremendously in their germination periods and their viability. In the one flower-head weeds have seeds that are programmed to germinate in twelve months' time, in three years' time and, in some cases, in ten years' time. They have little 'think-cells' that wait until their particular weather and climatic pattern arrive before they consent to germinate at all. Some of them travel miles on animals' coats or feet, are tramped round by humans on soles of shoes, are moved along by rain-water drainage, until they find appropriate settling positions; and, unlike most garden plants, the seeds germinate on the surface of the ground, not needing to be buried at all. So you can imagine the fighting power in roots that have to penetrate rocky railway-sidings or gravel-strewn roadsides, or barren pasturelands with their life-seeking threads. Weeds have roots that grow three to five times faster than the plant itself, burrowing down through topsoil and into subsoil with tremendous vitality and speed; opening up drainage channels so that the life-giving water can find its way to the roots; breaking up and conditioning hard subsoil. Some weeds actually exude chemical substances that break up soil structure.

Experimental work with weeds has gained in interest and importance as conservationists and the general population become more aware of the lack of fertility now so obvious in our soils. How do the weeds still grow? They cling on and fight for survival after every other wanted plant has given up. Imagine, then, what sources of natural chemicals and vitamins and minerals must be in such sturdy, resistant, vital plants. Most of our knowledge of herbal medicine has sprung from simple folk-remedies, from country people who used local weeds for their health-restoring properties. Most of the herbs classified in botanical encyclopaedias are in some part of the world a common weed growing in the open or amongst cultivated crops, growing in forests and waste areas. Hybridised plants (with the accent perhaps on magnificent flowers or leaf colouring) are like inbred people; their sturdy growth-stock has gradually weakened so that severe limitations are put upon their vitality and their capacity for survival is lost. That is why we have to coddle and pander to our prize roses and dahlias and chrysanthemums while the dandelions and buttercups and clovers are rampaging along at their feet. Those same prize roses must be grafted onto rootstock of the original wild rose to give them sufficient life to grow at all.

Weeds can teach us many lessons in survival as well as giving us natural, free greenstuff to use either as food or for simple medicines. There are goodies and baddies, of course. Don't go out and pick every plant along the roadside convinced that its life and chemicals will be good for you. There are some weeds and naturally occurring plants that can kill you very efficiently and very fast, some that can make you extremely ill, some that can give you diarrhoea and stomach-ache, depending on what they contain. One of the first things to do in learning about weeds and how they can help you is to know what weed is which. One student of mine, carried away completely by all that free food growing all over her block of virgin land, nibbled little bits of almost everything there, in particular a plant she described as having the most beautiful blue flowers. She was lucky: she merely had diarrhoea for a week.

With these naturally occurring plants, knowledge and discrimination are essential. If in any doubt whatsoever as to which plant it is that you have pulled up off the roadside (though you may think it is red dock, or wild carrot) send a specimen to your local Department of Agriculture or to your Botanic Garden experts for identification. For this you need a stem of the plant with, if possible, four to six leaves and one or more flowers, or one flower and a bud. It helps if you can also send a seed or seed-pod or seed-head. One little leaf from one little plant is not sufficient for a positive identification to be made, and it is in your own interests to be as painstaking as possible in the presentation of the specimen for classification.

Presuming that you have thus acquired the necessary knowledge, it is pleasant to think that you can walk along a roadside and pick some ingredients for a healthful salad, something to stop your mosquito bites itching, something to tone up your liver—and it's all free! When people ask me whether weeds grown along roadsides or on railway embankments, in park areas or nature strips, become polluted, my answer is an interesting academic one that explains why weeds can withstand fumes and smog and still flourish and flower and set seed. Most weeds have two different root systems, one that sends deep foraging roots on expeditions down into the soil, and a second system of fine rootlets and hair roots closer to the soil surface. The stronger foraging roots seek out minerals and foodstuffs in the subsoil; this nutriment is returned to the plant by osmosis and capillary action, and is processed by the fine surface-root system. In most cases the surface roots do little or no absorbing from the soil: they receive the raw materials from the deeper roots and fabricate them into plant food. So they are less affected by pollution in the air or in the top layers of soil than are other plants without this dual root system.

Weeds, therefore, have access to the heavier minerals and deep soil nutriment that other more cultivated plants, with their shorter life-span, do not possess: they have their own reservoirs of unpolluted, unchemicalised, untreated natural food deep down in the soil. Their exploring roots, diving down and burrowing their way, create not only paths for their own progress but drainage channels to loosen up soggy surface soil and to break up deep clay and mineral areas; and they also form closely connected pathways with the roots of other plants growing near to them. Thus they make available to these other plants the nutriment they bring up from low soil levels for themselves. Try leaving your weeds in a field of corn, not artificially planted but just growing naturally in amongst the corn; and grow another bed of corn close by that you keep carefully weeded. Carry out this experiment faithfully over one growing season and you will be astonished at the increased yield from the plot where the weeds are allowed to grow naturally. If you feel you must cut off the top-hamper growth of weeds, you can chop them a little and throw them straight back onto the ground to act as a natural mulch to give the soil surface protection from heat and evaporation.

You have been conditioned to think that a heavy crop of weeds will take away food and water from a cultivated crop growing with them. This is not usually the case, because not only do the weeds find their food elsewhere, down in the deeper soil layers, but they return deep soil water to the surface along their roots by capillary action, thus bringing water to the area where your cultivated crop can use it. You will not have to water or irrigate your crops so much if you allow a weed cover to grow in amongst them.

Nature has a lot to teach you about survival and growth and fertility, as you will find if you get out of the car on a week-end drive to observe the weeds at the roadside. Dig out a few little weed clumps here and there and look at the condition of the soil. See how much softer and easier it is to dig than the dirt that is bare of weeds at the road's edge. Dig a little deeper and see what else you can find out about the roots that are below; grub out some of those dense pockets of weed roots and see how strongly they have been feeding the plant to give it its life and strength. There could be, in one small patch, red dock and wild oat-grass, a dandelion or two, some creeping clover or the white-flowered heads of clover, varieties of grasses you've never seen before—all bound together and all having enough nutriment to stay alive and to thrive. It is an interesting property of weeds that they can grow in companionship with one another or with other plants to mutual benefit. Weed roots are not only compatible with but actually accompany roots of other compatible plants down through the soil, one root system closely following another, and both benefiting from the foodstuffs and water supply they discover. Now you know why the weed roots in your garden are so tenacious when you try to pull them up. Don't bother! Chop their tops off if their unkempt appearance troubles you, and allow the tremendous root systems to remain in the soil and gently rot away, leaving open drainage channels and air access to subsoil, so that bacteria and humus material will eventually penetrate into deeper soil layers, eliminating your need for a rotary hoe.

Many weeds replace nitrogen in the soil, just as legumes do, particularly in the deeper layers where nitrogen penetration is not usually high. You dig your garden not only to keep the soil clear of weeds and functioning well in a broken-up state, but to allow bacterial agents to penetrate and break up the more densely compacted subsoil. Give your aching back a rest and let the weeds do it for you. Nature ensures that her species survive by a process not only of natural selection but, in many cases, of mutual assistance. In Nature you seldom find one species of plant occupying an area alone. Plants that can benefit each other in their growth habits and their inter-dependent chemical exchange tend to grow together. The root systems of our cultivated plants have become used to receiving the majority of their food through the soil surface, by artificial means. We pour on liquid manure, we feed with superphosphate, we add trace minerals, and we water or irrigate from the soil surface, so that the plant has no need for its roots to go deeper to find nourishment. No one fertilises weeds. They therefore have to forage and hunt for their own food and to find ecological companions to help them. It is only when all seeds have been washed away together with the dust-like film of topsoil that weeds cannot reclaim and restore a soil that has been artificially denuded of life. The dustbowls created by drought following drought on artificially fed soils may appear irreclaimable; but if there are weed seeds there is still hope that a sudden wet season will lay the dust and germinate even a few of the long-term seeds that have waited, some of them for many years, until the right set of climatic conditions occurred to bring them to life.

Weeds can restore grass growth to pasturelands. Grass clumps demand surface friability, and while they are in good growth they maintain a sod-like condition of the top few centimetres of the soil. If for any reason this sod state is destroyed—by overgrazing, by extremes of drought that wither and bake the roots, by prolonged rains that rot them—grass does not have the type of root system able to recondition the soil for its regrowth unless weeds are there to start the process. Grass then has the ability to rout the weeds once its own growth conditions are available again. You might say weeds are the servitors of the plant kingdom: they do a lot of the hard work keeping the other plants alive. Pasturelands denuded of grass and taken over by natural weed growth have therefore the capacity to return to pasture again once climatic conditions are favourable. The weeds will disappear, having done their job.

The seeds found in most weed growth fall into two distinct categories: one type germinates when conditions are favourable to the plant's growth; the other germinates only when adverse conditions are present. As though it were highly imbued with the plant equivalent of adrenalin, the second type goes into action only when there is a struggle for survival.

Weeds are the cheapest and most readily available source of green manure. Hoe them out or chop them off at surface level if you must, and after they have been used as a mulch to retain moisture and to improve the surface texture gently turn them in: the fibrotic process of their degeneration will condition and strengthen the topsoil. Nature uses weeds to return to the soil surface the heavier minerals and elements that have trickled down to deeper levels beyond the reach of other plants. Capillary action will return some of the substances to the surface, but the process is greatly facilitated when weeds grow in the area. Weeds have their natural place in natural surroundings as a part of Nature's cycle; but there's little point in telling a botanic gardens' planner that he should have a small forest of nut-grass and onionweed and purslane and plantain flourishing amongst his display of brilliant roses and his formal stone pool edged with statues. If we want formal beauty we must employ gardeners not only to remove the weeds but to feed back into the soil the materials that would normally be available were the weeds present. I am not an advocate for lazy gardeners, but I am sure weeds have their place in many situations when fertility must be restored to soil, and when large areas of pastureland or food crops must be planted with the greatest economy and the least artificial help.

In my own herb garden I have found weed growth to be invaluable when I haven't enough time to care for my herb plants as I would wish. I can, when there is time, cultivate or compost, I can feed the plants with natural seaweed fertiliser, I can water them, I can mulch and cover the warm soil to retain heat in the winter and moisture in the summer; but I can't do it nearly as well as the weeds that have grown up there can do it for me. My herbs have never looked better since they have been left alone to form friendships with whatever weeds have sprung up in their vicinity. There is fleabane near thymes, there is clover running mad around the comfrey clump, and there are all sorts and conditions of other weeds naturally selecting their companion plants for mutual nourishment. I know that when I have the time to get into my garden again, removing weed growth and tidying up the edges and trimming and pruning and generally restoring to my herb garden some semblance of respectability, the plants will once more need feeding and watering and much more care. The weeds have been good caretakers for me in the meantime.

USEFUL WEEDS

Apart from their usefulness in the soil, some common weeds can be of considerable benefit to mankind.

Dandelions

We can start with a weed that is now world-wide in its distribution, the dandelion. Dandelions we have known from childhood when we blew away the seed-heads and watched their white fluffiness disintegrate into a thousand little arrow-shaped seeds borne off by the wind. The seed-heads must wait until the wind, or some child blowing at them, carries the seeds off to their next area of germination, where they will wait until conditions are right for their lives to begin.

Dandelion greens—the leaves of the dandelion—can be added to the vegetable content of our diet every day, for they have almost every element necessary to maintain healthy body function. They are rich in iron, in silicon, in magnesium, in sodium, and extremely rich in calcium; they contain potassium for the nervous system and the kidneys, phosphorus for maintaining healthy nerve function, sulphur as a body-cleansing agent, natural oxalic acid to cleanse gall and kidneys, and a high trace-mineral content as well. There is a high vitamin A content (14 000 units per hundred grams of leaves), vitamins B_1 and B_2, vitamin C, together with choline (the liver-regulating substance), and minimal amounts of thiamin and riboflavin. It seems almost too much to get from one simple plant. But the health-giving and therapeutic value of dandelion greens is beyond doubt, and they grow widely and abundantly.

There is only one snag: the so-called dandelions that grow wild and in abundance on pasturelands are not dandelions at all. The true dandelion plant has several distinguishing features, and it is most important that you recognise these before you pick anything that you hope will contain all the virtues of dandelion. True dandelions grow in a pale-green rosette of leaves, without hairs or spines or spikes of any kind: these leaves are soft and yellowish-green and deeply indented or toothed in several different corrugated patterns. Some dandelions have only four or five indentations per leaf, others have up to twenty; but they all share the distinguishing characteristics of no hairs and soft green leaves. The true dandelion also can be distinguished when in flower by the fact that each flower is borne on a single stem.

There is a plant masquerading as a dandelion, with indubitably dandelion-type flowers, which has a dark-green rosette of leaves lying flat against the ground, these leaves being slightly hairy and glossy, and the flower stems are borne on tall, branching stalks with many flowers in a candelabra effect. This is not a dandelion. Many people have used this plant in the belief that it was a dandelion, and have had no health benefit from it—except that they have been getting fresh greens. Remember, the real dandelion has no hairs, it has a leaf that is soft and not shiny, and each flower is borne on a single pale green stem.

Dandelion greens are used extensively in Europe and North America as a standard green vegetable and are chopped into the salad bowl as well. Their slightly bitter taste mingled with other salad greens is scarcely noticeable—if it bothers you at all. I would never cook a dandelion leaf if I could eat it raw, following the natural law that each processing step with a food reduces its vitality and its benefit to the body. Fresh dandelion leaves picked an hour or two before you intend to eat them give you the maximum benefit.

The root of the dandelion is roasted to provide the basis for making dandelion coffee. A daily ration of this beverage is recommended for anyone who has had liver complaints (such as hepatitis) or who suffers from a liver weakness. Dandelion coffee can be taken as a preventive measure, to ensure that the liver is strengthened and restored to its peak efficiency and that it remains healthy enough to be immune to invading bacterial or viral infections.

Dandelion greens are highly alkaline in their body reaction, and therefore indicated for arthritic sufferers, and as a corrective measure for people addicted to beer and white bread. They are completely digested within two and a half hours, and their tonic action on liver and kidneys alone is enough to put them high on every list of salad vegetables. Leave the roots in the soil, just whip off those soft green leaves, and before a week or so has passed, new top growth will be there for you to use again.

Dock and Sorrel

Another useful world-wide weed is dock, sometimes called red dock, and its cousin sorrel in all its various forms. All the sorrel family contain a good balance of minerals: calcium, potassium, chlorine and iron, with lesser amounts of phosphorus and sodium, plus an exceptionally high content of sulphur for a green-leafed vegetable. This is why they can have such a tonic effect on the bloodstream. The organic sulphur cleanses the body of waste accumulations, a process helped by sorrel's high vitamin A content (nearly 13 000 international units for every hundred grams of sorrel), thus taking weight off the liver and providing it with the vitamin A so essential to its correct function. Sorrel is also exceedingly high in vitamin C and is, like dandelion, quick to digest.

Dock and sorrel contain oxalic acid, and over and over again I hear the tale about the harm vegetables rich in oxalic acid can do. I assure you that *natural* oxalic acid can be handled by the body with no excess build-up into gallstones, kidney stones, bladder stones or any other type of calcification, unless other predisposing factors are present. Oxalates, the basic material comprising stone formation in the body, can be built up from many different sources; but natural oxalic acid does not necessarily contribute to their formation at all.

It can have quite the opposite effect, cleansing the blood-stream altogether, removing free calcium and converting it into substances more readily assimilated.

Horehound

Horehound is another common weed that can have tremendous value when properly understood and applied. There are two types, the white and the black horehound, so called because one has whitish furry leaves and the other has darker, green ones, but both have the typical horehound flower, rosettes of prickly seeds encircling a long papery stem. These seeds adhere to the wool of sheep and sometimes to the hair and hide of grazing cattle, and are transported from pasture to pasture.

Because of their high vitamin C content, horehound leaves are used medicinally for colds and flu and for many chest complaints involving congestion and infection. Horehound contains a bitter principle, marrubin, and a lot of sodium as well as vitamin C. You can chew eight to ten leaves of horehound twice a day if you live in an area where it grows, and you will know that you have had your vitamin C supplement. Horehound may be more palatable if you chop the leaves and mix them with a little honey to offset the extremely bitter, astringent flavour. If sufferers from bronchitis and chronic lung infections eat horehound as part of their daily diet they can banish, without any cost, many of the destructive processes going on in lungs and bronchial tree.

Marshmallow and Malva

I remember my mother brewing up a concoction of marshmallow and malva, together with beeswax and a little honey, which we used as a treatment for teenage acne, rubbing the cooled ointment on the skin externally, and internally taking a brew made from the marshmallow roots and leaves and the malva leaves as well. Now I know why she did it and why it was so effective: malva contains up to 17 per cent of essential minerals and has one of the highest vitamin A counts of any herb—approximately 268 000 units of vitamin A per 500 grams. Marshmallow contains a variety of good things, all of which are useful in purifying the bloodstream, balancing the nervous system, and supplying essential minerals to a body coping with puberty, which is when acne usually occurs at its highest level. It contains pectin, iron, albumin, asparagin for kidney function, lecithin for nervous function and blood-vessel elasticity, enzymes, mallic acid and 7 per cent of mineral ash which is very rich in phosphates. What better combination of free, readily available weeds could you get to treat and soothe not only the physical but the emotional trauma connected with acne?

Watercress

I know of a freshly running stream in the foothills of the Blue Mountains area near Sydney where I can pick as much fresh natural watercress as time allows me. Watercress I have dealt with elsewhere, but its official standing is still that of a naturally occurring weed, so I shall say a little about it here. Watercress is another of Nature's free bonus extras to those who know enough to take advantage of the offer. One could live on fresh water and watercress for quite a considerable time if no other foodstuff was available. It has most of the necessary minerals, and is particularly high in iron and sulphur. (When sulpha drugs are prescribed by the medical profession for low-grade infections and stubborn streptococcal invasion, you can just eat watercress.) It is highly alkaline, and it tastes magnificent. You can toss it with a little oil and garlic and lemon and make a green salad fit to grace any table; or you can just pick it out of the stream, wash it thoroughly, and eat it raw and still living.

Watercress, together with nasturtiums and garden cresses of many descriptions, has 'antibiotic' properties similar to those of the onion family, and can be used for protection from colds and flu and in the treatment of chronic congestive illnesses. Nasturtium leaves, and the flowers too, always graced our Sunday-evening salad bowl when I was a child, the flowers giving exotic splendour and the green leaves their clean peppery taste to mingle with radishes and cucumber and whatever else my mother had growing in the garden. If you know of a naturally occurring clump of nasturtiums (and sometimes people dig them out of gardens and throw them on rubbish heaps or waste ground where they germinate readily and self-sow themselves for many seasons afterwards), raid the nasturtium patch for an extra-special salad.

Plantains

Another common weed can be useful in several simple health measures: the small plantain, *Plantago lanceolata*, sometimes called 'lamb's tongue'. This weed grows in almost every conceivable crack and cranny side by side with dandelions and small grasses, and as a child I used the pointed flower stem-heads as missiles, curling the stalk round in a loop behind the flower-head to fire them at other five-year-olds. This little weed has, like its larger plantain relatives, a particular use in cleansing the bloodstream and acting as a mild tonic. It is often added to so-called green drinks made from common weeds and vegetable material to give chlorophyll and plant minerals and vitamins to health-conscious juice addicts. I know a very hale and hearty sixty-five-year-old farmer, an orchardist, who mixes himself a green drink every morning from many different weeds and herbs growing wild around his property. Another ingredient he uses as often as possible is red clover, *Trifolium pratense*, the stuff that Walt Disney's rabbits always eat in glorious Technicolor.

Red Clover

Red clover is an interesting medicinal herb as well as a common pasture weed, being extremely rich in iron and copper and therefore useful in many diseases based on malfunction of the circulation. It has even been used for whooping cough and many assorted ills where other herbs and weeds either react slowly or do not give positive benefit. You can make a magnificent tea from either fresh or dried red clover flower-heads and a few top leaves from each stem: unlike other herb teas this one should be boiled for at least five minutes, so that all the iron and copper are extracted from the plant. We are not looking for vitamin content here, so the boiling does not detract from the medicinal value of the plant; we are only seeking those two vital minerals. How much better, though, to have your red clover in full delicate bloom straight off the ground from under the apple-trees and pear-trees where this healthy farmer plucks his. I have spent time on his orchard and come home feeling so full of health and vitality that I can only agree with his green-drink therapy. You have not lived until you have picked red, firm apples straight from the tree and eaten them mouthful by mouthful alternating with some of the weeds growing round the tree's sturdy base. There was plantain there too, and wild oat-grass and several other species of clover, together with another interesting herb called locally fat hen or lamb's quarter. The roots of this plant, *Chenopodium album*, dive deeply into subsoil, and it is rich in minerals and trace elements and vitamins. My friend the farmer used the leaves not only in his green drink in the morning but for his midday salad, too. He threw in the hard little ears of wild oat-grass, *Avena fatua*, as well for its high natural silica content and roughage, and a few leaves of yellow-flowered wood sorrel, *Oxalis corniculata*, to round off his green salad.

Fennel

There are several introduced plants that are well on the way to becoming major weeds, and it's lucky for us that they are here and that they are rapidly covering as much ground as possible in the areas where they have found suitable growing conditions. One of these hardy weeds flourishes along railway lines and roadsides and riverbanks, flowering yellow and tall and feathery around early January, and setting a multitude of aromatic seeds on its umbrella-shaped heads later in February and March. This is fennel, *Foeniculum vulgare*, a beautiful weed not only for general health but for culinary delights as well. Fennel seeds give their characteristic aniseed flavour to bortsch soup, the classic Russian beetroot brew, as well as adding piquancy to bread-rolls and cakes and perking up cottage cheese for your midday salad. Gather all the wild fennel seeds you can when they are ripe (they will be mid to darkish brown in colour by then) and store them in an airtight glass jar for your next twelve months' supply. Seeds from these wild fennel plants have much more flavour and value than those from garden or cultivated fennel, and can be stored without losing their viability and freshness for anywhere up to ten years. Don't use the wild fennel stems or leaves for your salads, though, or you will spend a lot of time and effort munching fibrous material approximately of the consistency of sugar-cane. Wild fennel becomes very stringy in its stems and leaves, so the garden variety is better to use in your salad. Fennel seeds can be nibbled in between meals to allay hunger, which they do very effectively; or they can be used instead of a meal if you wish to control excess weight caused by over-eating or compulsive eating.

Chicory

Chicory, *Cichorium intybus*, is the second of these valuable imported plants now growing in weed profusion amongst pastures and along roadside ditches and banks—to the benefit of any cattle grazing in the area, and to the delight, when they are in flower, of passers-by. The tall, cathedral spires of blue flowers, carried on branching stems, open very early in the morning in their brilliant deep blue, and fade as sunlight gathers intensity to a soft grey by about mid-afternoon. They could be a gardener's delight, as well as a farmer's friend and everybody's liver tonic.

Chicory is similar to dandelion in its physical properties,

the youngish leaves being almost interchangeable with dandelion in both chemical constituency and taste. As the plant matures, the leaves disappear and the flower spike shoots up to its full height of 120 to 150 centimetres (4 to 5 feet); so if you want your chicory for medicinal purposes grab it while it's young. Chicory, as you know, can be mixed with coffee, and some commercial preparations are still available in which it is added to coffee essence. This is a great way to take your coffee if you flatly refuse to give it up altogether, because the chicory mitigates—to a certain extent, anyway—the harmful effects of coffee on your liver. There is not enough chicory in the mixture to make it a health drink by any means, but at least you are helping your liver to tolerate the coffee.

Chickweed

Chickweed, *Stellaria media*, is a useful, soft-leaved, soft-stemmed inconspicuous tenant of many weed patches, and you may have to search a little to find it. Its pale-green floppy stems trailing untidily over the soil surface are fragile and can be pulled off easily to chop into your salad, or to use as poulticing material to draw out infections or foreign bodies through the skin. Make yourself a chickweed poultice with a small handful of leaves and stems: Wash them, then heat them in as little water as possible to bring them only to blood temperature. Pack the sloshy material over a boil or a carbuncle that you want to draw to the surface, or indeed over any skin eruption that needs to suppurate. You can draw out splinters with this poultice, or a sliver of glass, or a piece of metal; and it is useful when any foreign matter pierces the eye—such a delicate spot—and needs to be extracted without damaging the tissues. Packed over the eyelids, it will gently draw any foreign body as it soaks deep through the lids and into the membranes of the eyeball itself. It is useful in conjunctival infections when irritation and grittiness are felt behind the lids themselves, easing the irritability and drawing out any foreign matter causing it. Chickweed ointment is

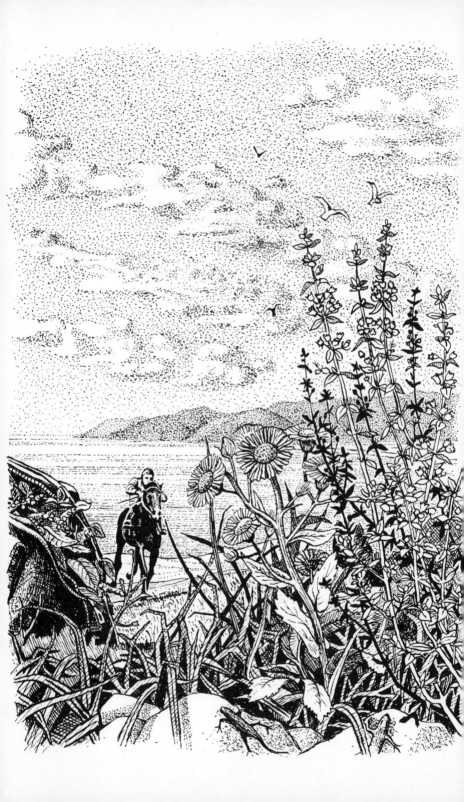

available from health stores under its botanical name of Stellaria Media, and can be kept in the medicine cupboard for any emergencies when you cannot get fresh chickweed.

Do not confuse chickweed and milkweed. Milkweed has white, sappy stems often used by country folk to treat skin conditions of many types—from warts to skin cancer. The sap from milkweed is so caustic during the spring and summer months, its maximum growth period, that it will burn off any growths on the surface of the skin; but it can also burn deeper still and leave you with a raw, weeping area of exposed epidermis. Leave milkweed severely alone unless you have weather-worn skin like old leather, which will not mind if the top few layers are completely removed. Many a farmer and his family using milkweed have probably been saved from severe skin problems because constant exposure has hardened their skins.

Couch-grass

Do you know you can chop up the couch-grass runners that straggle into your flower-beds and put them in the salad bowl, too? *Agropyron repens*, or English couch-grass as we know it in lawns, is a good tonic and stimulatory cleanser for the kidneys. Small amounts of its white runner-roots (not the hair rootlets dropping down into the soil from them) can be eaten from time to time: but certainly not every day or you will wear a very deep track to your bathroom.

Castor-oil Plant

The castor-oil plant, *Ricinus communis*, grows and flourishes on waste ground, particularly if it can get its roots into moisture or marshy conditions. You will know its large umbrella-shaped green leaves and thick, hollow, bamboo-like stalks, growing from 10 to 12 feet (300 to 360 centimetres) in height, with the typical reddish tinge on some of the leaves and the round spiky balls of green or red clustered on the flowering stem and later turning to the seed-pod. Here is a weed that can be dangerous, particularly since its bright colours seem to have an attraction for small children. When the seed-pods are ripe they burst open and throw the seed away from the plant, ensuring its spread into clumps and groves and whole paddocks if the soil is hospitable. Two of these black seeds, if eaten, can be enough to cause severe diarrhoea and stomach cramps, and a small child could quickly be in a critical condition. So let us keep the castor-oil plant at a safe distance and merely consider the qualities of the oil we need not attempt to extract for ourselves. Forget about taking castor oil—that purgative beloved of our grandmothers—if the very thought of it is repugnant to you: there are plenty of other good aperients. A gentler way to make use of the oil's virtues is to apply it externally as a poultice to draw inflammation and irritation and even infection from the body via the skin.

Warm a little castor oil (a couple of tablespoons is plenty) and before applying it to any skin area test it with your elbow or with your finger to make sure that it is at blood heat only. Smear the warm oil thoroughly over the affected area, cover with brown paper or with an old piece of sheeting, and make the patient (it may be yourself) lie about for an hour or two while the oil does its drawing out through the skin. Castor oil, as you probably know, has a sticky and very penetrating action on clothing as well as skin, so don't lie on the best chair or sofa. If possible, it is best to let the oil poultice do its work out in the warm sun. This treatment can ease severe bronchitic infections, particularly in young children; but see that the patient, young or old, is kept thoroughly warm on a cool day.

Castor oil will remove foreign bodies, such as splinters, slivers of glass or bee stings, as well as drawing out boils and carbuncles. It is also useful for fungoid inflammations and infections such as whitlows (paronychia) with its penetrating, gentle action. It can be used safely to remove foreign bodies from the eye. Smear castor oil liberally under the eyelids where it will gently form a film and draw and soothe while floating offending material to the surface and out along natural channels at a natural speed. The eyes may be very sticky and gummy the next morning, but the irritation and the foreign bodies should be well and truly gone. The soles of the feet are particularly vulnerable when young and old prefer to go barefooted, and castor oil can safely and gently remove anything that has penetrated and lodged deeply in the hardened soles. Poultice the area with warm oil and leave the poultice, preferably overnight, to draw and soften the hard, keratosed skin. (I have used chickweed interchangeably with castor oil.) With such poulticing I was able to remove from my son's foot a sea-urchin spine embedded well below the surface and ignored by him until his toe swelled to twice the size and was too painful to put to the ground.

Purslane

Purslane, *Portulaca sativa*, is a common weed in most gardens during the heat of summer. Its fleshy bright-green opposite leaves on reddish stems are a useful addition to a bowl of green salad when many other salad greens are scarce. It is a relative of the garden portulaca, the showy, sun-loving annual that grows and flowers about the same time. Purslane, like borage, can have a distinctly cooling effect in the body, and its high alkalinity is good for acid stomachs. It has a pleasant astringent taste; but it's better to use only the leaves for your salad.

Seaweed

Kelp, whose other name is seaweed, is just that: a sea weed instead of a land one. It is free, it is available, and it is a magnificent source of vitamins and minerals. There are hundreds and hundreds of seaweeds and you should have the knowledge to pick the good from the bad. Although most of them have no harmful effects whatsoever, there are some better left to be eaten by snails or fish.

Three of the good ones are bladderwrack, *Fucus vesiculosus*, one of the seaweeds commonly lumped together and called kelp; agar agar, *Gelidium amansil*, a useful little seaweed that can be boiled to produce a neutral-tasting jelly as a base for many sweets and savoury dishes; and Irish moss, *Chondrus crispus*, which is somewhat similar. If you are game, you can walk around at low tide amongst the rock pools, soaking up your ration of sunshine and salt from natural sources and clear sea air, and nibbling at bits of this and that. In general it is wiser to leave red, blue or purple seaweeds alone. Some of them are safe and some of them are not, and it's best to take no risks.

Sea lettuce, *Ulva latucea*, a green seaweed beloved of sea snails and crustaceans, can be eaten in moderation by humans too. The Japanese and Chinese and Eastern nations know very well the dietary benefits of many different kinds of seaweed. They use it in dried form; they powder it and grind it; some use it fresh. They know well its value for the soil as well as for them, spreading it on farmland and gardens where its trace elements and heavy minerals replace those leached out by rain-water run-off and intensive soil cultivation. There are so many different kinds of edible seaweed that I cannot describe and classify them all. If you are in doubt, send a specimen of the seaweed to your Marine Biology Department for classification, and ask whether it has proved to be safe and edible.

Wild Strawberry

The hybridised large red fruits of the cultivated strawberry we all know and eat as often as our income allows; but did you know that the wild strawberry, *Fragaria vesca*, has more than five times the dietary value of its better-bred cousin? The fruits of the wild strawberry contain iron in an easily assimilable state, and their leaves, like raspberry leaves, have been used to correct menstrual problems and to prevent natural abortion, for they are high in folic acid and contain tonic properties for muscles in the pelvic area.

Wild Raspberry

The wild raspberry plant seems to withstand disease, especially mosaic disease, considerably better than the cultivated variety, so if you want to drink raspberry-leaf tea pick the wild leaves if possible.

The leaves of wild raspberry contain a substance called fragrane, which, though not yet fully analysed, appears to have a marked effect on the female organs of reproduction, especially on the muscles of the pelvic region and the uterus. It has been prescribed from the earliest months of pregnancy to counteract morning sickness and to act as a tonic medicine so that the birth will be as simple, painless and natural as possible; its secondary use is to alleviate afterbirth pains and help in expelling the placenta. Raspberry leaves have also been prescribed for sterility in both male and female when lack of muscle tone in the reproductive organs is thought to be the cause. A cupful of raspberry-leaf tea can be taken every morning during pregnancy without any fears of its harming mother or child. Like carrots or lettuce or celery, it has tonic and strengthening properties.

Did you know that the stains on your fingers after a wild-berry-gathering expedition can be removed very simply by rubbing one or two of the green, unripe crushed berries of the same plant over the stained area? When your children go gathering mulberries or blackberries or raspberries, tell them to bring home some of the unripe berries as well. A little diligent rubbing will remove all stains from skin and clothing.

Blackberries

Blackberries, *Rubus fruticosus*, which grow in civilised fashion in colder countries, tend to romp in abandoned proliferation where the climate is warmer. Our diligent pest-control and weed-control authorities chop down the blackberry clumps and spray them mightily with brown clouds of defoliant or some other burning-type corrosive poison that scorches them brown and stops growth for a limited period. If you are fortunate enough to know where there is a stand of wild blackberries, unsprayed, unpoisoned, and growing vigorously and densely, keep an eye on them until the fruit is ripe then eat as many as you can of the ripe berries. They will make you sleep well, and improve your bowel habits, and cool and condition your bloodstream and circulatory system. I spent a happy afternoon with friends on their country property by the river picking organically grown unsprayed tomatoes, and alternating my frequent sampling of the ripe, sweet, magnificent fruit with handfuls of blackberries growing unchecked along the side fences. You have never tasted tomatoes until you have picked them richly vermilion and full of juice and sweetness straight from the plant, then counteracted their bittersweet bite with a handful of dark, mineral-rich blackberries.

Nettles
When you brush against the stinging nettle, *Urtica dioica*, you give a sudden yelp and have a lot of itching skin for one, two, or three days afterwards. I had a brush with stinging nettles that was an education for me both physically and botanically when, having tried to import into my herb gardens small plants of stinging nettles that miserably died, I found in the Snowy Mountains area of New South Wales stinging nettles of an entirely different breed. They grew in dense thickets around clear streams that ran fast and pure from the high glacial basins between the mountains. Most of them were above my shoulder, flourishing gigantically as the mineral-rich waters from the snows poured down, feeding them with the minerals and moisture they absorbed through the almost black depths of the natural compost where they grew. My walking shoes sank, sometimes above the ankle, into an

organic stew such as those poor struggling little nettle plants in my garden would never know.

On that walking trip we had to clamber down through one patch of nettles to get to water each night, then up through another patch the next morning to find a ridge and pursue our course. I shall never forget the state of my hands and face after battling through these dense thickets of nettle: I was scratched and bleeding and red-raw from the irritating poisons in the nettle barbs along each stem and leaf. Luckily I was carrying with me a little pot of herbal ointment made from—guess what?—nettles. As with many plants in herbal medicine, small quantities of the plant cure what the plant itself causes. Nettle is often prescribed in ointment form for bee stings, for ant stings and bites, for tick bites, even for mosquito bites and fly bites, and for any skin irritation caused by plants to which the sufferer is sensitive. My nettle ointment reduced the severity of the stings and also the irritation and inflammation of the cuts and scratches.

Stinging nettles have tremendous health value used as a cooked green, or medicinally as prescribed by herbalists and naturopaths. The fresh green nettle tips can be picked (using gloves, of course), and steamed like any other green vegetable to give a daily ration of iron and copper, as well as calcium, lecithin for the blood-vessel walls and the nervous system, and sodium and potassium and chlorine in a natural balanced state. The vitamin A content of nettle is not destroyed by the boiling and is then available to benefit skin, liver, and other organs as well as metabolic processes.

In olden times nettles were made into bunches and used as flails to beat the deadened, wasted limbs of patients suffering from muscular atrophy, wasting, and paralysis. The nerve-irritating poison in the spines stimulated the peripheral nerves and blood vessels, restoring some circulation and nerve supply.

Nettles have also been used to restore hair growth to a bald head. If baldness is the result of insufficient blood supply to the hair follicles and roots, or if circulation has been impeded in the scalp area by dandruff or cradle cap or psoriasis, treatment with nettles would certainly restore function to the skin. And there is no need to beat the patient's head with a bunch of nettles: make a pot of nettle tea from the dried leaves—or from the fresh leaves if you have a nettle patch growing near you—and use this as a final rinse when washing the hair. If you are totally bald, presumably you don't wash your hair; but nettle has produced regrowth of hair in total baldness if faulty circulation and insufficient nerve supply to the scalp has been the predisposing cause. Many hair tonics and shampoos contain nettle, and these are undoubtedly stimulating to the whole scalp area.

Maidenhair

While we are on the subject of hair, there is another freely growing wild plant, the maidenhair fern, *Adiantum capillus-veneris*, which can be made into a tea and used as a rinse for toning the hair. Pick a good handful of the leaves growing wild in damp corners of woodland and pour a cup or so of boiling water over them, then leave the brew to stand for an hour or so, strain, and rub well into the scalp.

Stay away from any wild plants or weeds that have bright orange or bright green berries until you have been given an accurate classification of the plants and know whether they are edible or whether they could be harmful to you. Many plants with orange berries have acid properties that can be not only caustic but corrosive if taken internally or rubbed into the skin.

Mullein

Mullein, *Verbascum thapsus*, is a common weed from Europe and North America that is rapidly spreading in the Snowy Mountains area of Australia. It is a beautiful plant with greyish blanket-like leaves growing in a large rosette and a spike of pale primrose flowers growing from the centre; and at Christmas-time it is found up and down the roadsides and spreading into cow pastures and paddocks. Cattle eating the flowers of mullein are doing themselves a lot of good, as well as clearing the roadside of what many people consider a weed. Another name for mullein is cow lungwort. It acts on the lungs and is prescribed in herbal remedies for asthma, bronchitis, and any form of lung infection and congestion. Make a herb tea from the leaves and flowers of the plant. A good-sized handful is usually enough for each cup, and you pour boiling water on it in the usual way, let it stand for an hour, then strain and drink a small cupful both night and morning. The steam from the hot mullein brew can also be inhaled while you're waiting for it to cool sufficiently to drink. Just hang your head over the saucepan and let the fumes penetrate down to your lungs. If you wish to store the dry flowers and leaves, you must put them, after drying, in tins rather than in glass jars, for they turn black if exposed to the light.

Paterson's Curse

An Australian *bad* weed, with close relatives in most parts of the world, is *Echium plantagineum*, known locally as Paterson's Curse or Salvation Jane. Graziers and farmers, as they watch its brilliant blue and purple canopy of flower-heads racing across paddocks during the summer months, call it by unprintable names. Its British relative, *Echium vulgare*, viper's bugloss, has been used in herbal medicine in chest and throat complaints. The Australian species has a nasty reputation for poisoning cattle and sheep. It contains in all parts of the plant an alkaloid that is thought to be the poisonous factor, but accurate reports of cases of poisoning are rare. Anyway, in case of doubt, chuck it out.

I was once given three little plants of what I was told was burdock, a valuable medicinal herb long used in European medicine in the treatment of arthritis, and I gave these plants an honoured placed in my herb garden, nurturing them and caring for them as a rarity that I had been anxious to obtain for a long time. As the plants grew, the basal rosette of leaves flourished mightily and up came the flowering stem right on time in the very early days of summer. Now I took a closer look at my 'burdock' and found it was certainly not burdock at all: it was in fact a fine little stand of Paterson's Curse! I let it flower just to be sure, and even by doing so I let it beat me, for the seeds set so rapidly and fell so prolifically that I have been digging out the plants from my herb garden ever since. Those original plants dropped time-release seeds, and every year just a few plants have grown from the seed that fell four and a half years earlier. I do not know of any obvious use for Paterson's Curse; but perhaps, apart from looking beautiful, it has some not-yet-discovered benefit to give us.

Privet

Another enemy among weeds is the common privet, *Ligustrum vulgare*. In cool climates it is a tame hedging plant, kept within bounds by determined gardeners with sharp shears; but in warmer climates it has become a rampant, noxious-weed shrub that can grow quickly into a tall tree. And how it spreads!—particularly if it has been cut when in berry and thrown onto waste ground. The poorer the soil and the harder the conditions the more it seems to thrive. In middle spring come its white flowers, loading the bush with a beautiful scented feathery cloak that drives hay-fever and asthma sufferers to drink, drugs and absolute misery. The berries of the privet can cause severe diarrhoea if eaten—particularly by young children, who seem attracted to the purplish-black clusters of privet berries often within their reach. These berries, and possibly the leaves too, contain a glycoside that can cause severe gastro-enteritis. There are records of horses and sheep having fatal attacks, so that the privet is now seldom planted as a hedge where livestock have access to it.

You can do your bit towards making life easier for the hay-fever brigade in your district by chopping down, or asking your local councils to chop down, any stands of privet before they come into flower. Councils have many odd jobs to do for ratepayers; but privet is a declared noxious weed in many parts of this country and you will surely get action. You have only to see the inflamed, congested, running eyes, the puffy red nose and swollen antrums of a real hay-fever sufferer to want to do your bit in removing privet before it flowers. If you really want to have it growing, keep it clipped and contained within formal bounds to stop its flowering altogether.

Bracken

The common bracken fern, *Pteridium aquilinum*, is a prolific wild plant. It grows on hillsides, amongst tall timber, on rocky barren ground, on wasteland. Indeed, when it has once commenced to grow it will spread and spread anywhere if conditions are right for it, until very little else can grow near it because its light-stealing canopy inhibits other weed growth beneath it. Bracken fern, particularly the rhizome or fleshy root, but also the leaves and stems as well, contain thiaminase and several other poisonous agents of doubtful chemical composition which can produce symptoms very much like those of vitamin B_1 deficiency in both man and animals. Cattle who regularly have nothing to eat but bracken show damage in the bone marrow; but mostly this poisoning takes place only when the bracken plant is young and green, its action being very much less and almost negligible when the plant is dried. Animals instinctively avoid eating anything harmful or potentially harmful to them, and eat bracken only if no other fodder at all is to be had.

Bracken has one very good use amongst all its dangerous qualities: the nests of the fighting bulldog-ants, those brown and black and green and yellow antediluvian monsters that abound in dry timber forests and eucalypt bush, are often tunnelled out amongst the strong deep roots and surface rhizomes of bracken fern. If you are stung by a bulldog-ant, look about you quickly for a *young* stem of bracken fern, break it carefully in the fleshiest part, and squeeze as much of the juice as you can onto the skin where the sting penetrated. It will act as a counter-irritant, alleviating the pain and to some extent inhibiting the swelling and itching that can follow.

WE'VE A LOT TO LEARN

There are hundreds of thousands of weeds that have not been analysed for their chemical constituents or investigated for their qualities. If you know of any local plants that perhaps your grandma used for her gout, or Uncle Ted used for baldness, or Cousin Milly vowed cured her sinusitis, let someone know about them (preferably me) so that they can be examined to determine their possible usefulness to man.

The way to discovering yet another plant that may be beneficial to man, or livestock, or the soil itself, is a long and arduous one. If a plant is suspected of being useful in some way, it must first be identified; then research must be done to discover whether it is mentioned in botanical writings, in pharmacognosy papers, in old herbal-medicine manuscripts; then inquiries have to be made as to whether any other researchers are conducting their own investigations into the same plant. That is only the beginning. The task the dedicated researcher must then undertake can be dangerous and even deadly if he or she is dedicated sufficiently: It is necessary to eat quantities of the plant, either its leaves or its roots or its flowers, and tabulate whatever clinical effects are observed. Whether it gives you fierce headaches or violent nausea or an itching rash, there is no other initial way to discover its effects and whether it is worth subsequent investigation. Much of the present-day knowledge of plant drugs was obtained in just this empirical way by brave or perhaps foolhardy individuals. It is entirely on your own head if you wish to go out and eat a particular plant to discover some of its properties; but unless you are trained in this field I would say it was highly inadvisable for you to do so.

The Chinese have their herbs and the North American Indians have theirs, and so do the Europeans and the Maoris and even the Eskimos. Every country should know as much as possible about its indigenous or introduced herbs, the weeds and herbs that can help so much with health, soil fertility and the growth of livestock and crops. And there is still much to be learnt in Australia.

Every showy garden hybrid perfected and birth-controlled until the exact colour and shape of its petals, the size of its blooms, and the extent of its reproduction can be ascertained, was once derived from a simple, natural wild growing plant. Weeds are the common ancestor, and their strength and vitality and resistance have ensured that our planet retains its topsoil and its oxygen exchange rate with a minimum of work from us. Take a second look at weeds and wild plants and be thankful they have minds of their own and survival instincts that keep them growing under the most adverse conditions. You can spray weed patches, you can burn them, you can soak their roots with hormone preparations, you can cultivate and bury them; you can take every conceivable destructive measure against them and next season that patch of ground will be covered with some sort of weed or other. It may not be the original one you set out to destroy, but you may have unwittingly provided conditions where the next weed in the cycle can take hold and give its contribution to retaining or regaining lost life in that particular weed patch. Learn from weeds some of the biological and natural lessons of survival that man may yet have to employ to ensure that his own species continues on this earth.

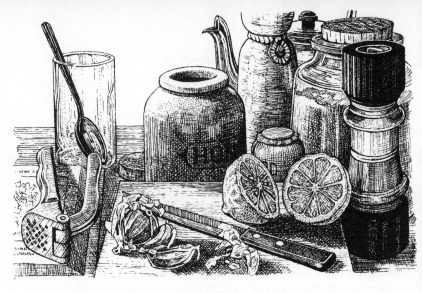

7

Simple Home Remedies
for Everyday Ills

THE COMMON COLD

The common cold is still withstanding all the technical discoveries and modern know-how of orthodox medicine: So far nothing has been found to 'cure' the common cold. It must be endured, with a multitude of pills, lotions and soothing drinks to help you feel better while it runs its course.

Here's a revolutionary approach to it for you: the common cold is not a disease at all! Naturopathic medicine holds the view that a cold is the first attempt by the body to throw off an approaching state of ill-health. Think of all the symptoms that appear when you have a cold: your nose is stuffy and clogged up with mucus, your head aches, your throat may be sore, dry and swollen, you may have a cough that hurts your chest or brings up phlegm, you will feel miserable and depressed, and your limbs and muscles move only at half speed.

Let's analyse these symptoms from a natural point of view.

Why is your nose choked and sore, and then running copiously from one or both nostrils? The mucous membranes lining the nasal passages are reacting with their own defences against attack by harmful agents like bacteria (streptococcal infection in particular), and they secrete more and more mucus to repel these attacks. Your body's control system has sensed a weakened area in the nasal passages where disease can strike and has put up its first line of defence, the only way Nature knows how—attack! Your swollen, choked-up nose is fighting hard, attempting to throw out of the body with the expelled mucus the harmful agents that are attacking it. Your throat is sore for the same reason: your body has felt an irritated area there (perhaps weakened by previous colds, laryngitis, tracheitis, or pharyngitis) and is repelling imminent attack by secreting mucus in the form of catarrh. You are constantly clearing your throat or feeling as if you want to. This is literally what you are doing—clearing the area of the attacking agents.

Why does your head ache? When any state of ill-health is approaching and sensed by the body, blood is rushed by it to the vital organs, giving them an increased supply of oxygen to burn out the invader and to stimulate the function of the tissues in the affected part. Your head aches not only from the pressure there of full sinuses and clogged antrums, but also because there is a slight increase in your blood pressure as it rushes supplies to the front-line troops. Your blood has to pump harder through the congested areas, and your head aches with the effort. Why do your limbs feel like lead and why are your muscles too weak to hold you upright? They are telling you—screaming at you, in fact—to stop and lie down as soon as you can, letting your body concentrate on strengthening itself sufficiently to be able to overcome the approaching state of ill-health. Why do you feel so depressed and miserable? Your nerves are also involved in this trouble, sensing pain and discomfort, and your glands are working overtime to surround and expel would-be attackers through the bloodstream and the other excretory channels like skin, bowels, and kidneys; and a sudden depression of the glandular responses results in mental depression as well. That cough you can't suppress during the quiet adagio passages at the symphony concert means that your body is still attempting to expel dangerous or potentially dangerous infecting agents from a weakened or vulnerable area.

The whole picture of the common cold is one of 'Repel boarders!' It is an acute defensive reaction to clear the ship. Most true colds run a course of several days in the acute phase, and if your vitality is high and your body responses strong, this can be the end of it. However, if a cold runs on and on and on, taking weeks to clear and never really leaving you, it is a sure sign that your body is not strong enough to throw off the next attack. This is not much consolation when you have a heavy cold. What you want is to know not why but *how* to stop feeling as you are feeling, how to get back to health again quickly.

A cold may now appear to you as something quite different from what it did before, but this is no good reason why you should have to endure it without help. This is where Nature comes in again, with simple, natural ingredients designed not to suppress the cold symptoms, as so many synthetic preparations do, but to help you fight off invaders.

Here is a natural recipe to help you when you have a cold— not to stop the processes that are going on but to give them more strength and speed. Buy a corm of garlic from your greengrocer and peel off one or two of the small cloves; crush them in your garlic press or with the flat edge of a large knife, having first removed the outer papery skin; then place them in a large heat-resistant tumbler. Squeeze the juice from a lemon and shred up some of the rind, too, if it's clean and fresh, and add this to the squashed garlic; then add about half a teaspoon of ground powdered ginger, then a pinch of cayenne pepper and, to top off the brew, a tablespoon of honey. Mix these ingredients, and add to them a cupful of water just off the boil. Drink the whole lot, solid as well as liquid if possible, as soon as it's bearably cool, and within ten to twenty minutes be in bed and covered up well. Here is what this fearsome concoction will do for you: The garlic is a powerful vegetable 'antibiotic', fighting off and inhibiting the growth and reproduction of bacteria such as the streptococcus. The lemon has an astringent, binding, contracting effect on the mucous membrane linings. The ginger acts on a stomach that can be irritated and upset by some of the catarrh and mucus from throat and nasal passages, first warming it, then increasing its blood supply and function as well as stimulating its secretory juices, and thus getting rid of the offending material as fast as possible into the bowel and out through the excretory channel. The pinch of cayenne pepper is just about right for a homoeopathic dose of vitamin C, one of the chief combatants on your side in this fight (homoeopathic quantities act in the body as a tiny trigger to start your own vitamin C working at top speed). Honey is the food of the gods—no doubt about that—but its use here is more earthly, as it soothes and heals all those red, raw tissue areas. This rather interesting-tasting concoction is aimed purely at hastening the body's excretory action. It will not suppress or inhibit any body process, but will boost along the body's natural immunity reaction. And why must you get into bed so fast? You will sweat profusely. The heat and the lemon and the garlic and the ginger and the cayenne will all produce strong excretory action through every channel possible: lungs, nose, skin and possibly bladder and bowel as well. If you have a bout of diarrhoea the next morning, praise the Lord! This means that your body has fought valiantly all night while you rested in sleep and has removed a large proportion of dangerous matter.

VIRUS INFECTIONS

We can't deal with so-called flu in quite the same fashion,

because its attacking agent is different and its methods of warfare really underhand. Viruses attack individual body cells and live either in them or partly in them, absorbing nutriment that the cells are thus deprived of—so they die. (This over-simplification of the biological process may help you to understand why you cannot 'kill' or remove the virus as easily as you can repel harmful bacteria.) There are many different compounds and drugs recommended by pharmaceutical companies that can most effectively remove the virus, but can also severely damage the cells that are hosts to the virus and are no longer functioning normally. This is why influenza can kill, and why it can leave traces of destruction in body tissues for many years or even a whole lifetime. When you have influenza you must realise that your body is in a serious state of siege.

Viruses may not be little green men from Mars, but they are a real threat to the animal kingdom, lying as they do half-way between being a vegetable and an animal themselves. I have seen patients showing signs in the iris of the eye (an area I use for diagnostic work) two, three and four years or more after having had a bout of viral influenza. Viruses don't know the rules applying to the rest of nature: They don't attack a weak area; they select as their host the strongest body cells, and you can see the sense of this from their point of view. The human cell has very little resistance naturally to virus entry, and the stronger the cell the more food and nutrition there is for the virus to live, grow and multiply. I am an optimist who believes that for every action there is a counterbalancing reaction, especially in the realm of survival. The key to the problem is there always; it's just a matter of finding which key opens the door. The organic acids found naturally in fruit and some vegetables have a discriminatory action on viruses. It's not that the viruses can't win: it's just that with knowledge and understanding we can't lose. If you have influenza (and how different it is from the common cold you will all know) go to bed, sip your pickle juice, eat plums, tomatoes or lemons if you feel like them; or wait until your body's maximum defence reaction has been mobilised in a high temperature to burn out whatever can be eliminated naturally, and then follow up with organic acids after the acute stage has passed. You can live very effectively for several days on water only while this initial acute phase is endured. Once the virus has been weakened by such treatment it can still, unfortunately, migrate to a more vulnerable site in the body, perhaps somewhere where previous structural or organic damage has taken place, and hibernate there, regrouping its forces for another attack. It's a sneaky little creature, biding its time until all the conditions are favourable once again.

In my experience, you are less likely to get flu if you can maintain your body at an optimum constant temperature. Sudden chills can bring to life viruses that have lain dormant for months or even years; so keep warm in the wintertime, when the danger of chilling is greatest. I had a lovely strong, healthy female patient who made one fatal mistake last winter when she took off for a day's sailing without warm gear. In a wet, miserable southerly gale, she was chilled to the bone for several hours, and the next morning she had the flu. I had seen in her iris on previous occasions the sign telling me that viral infection was a possibility in the lung and bronchial area; but while she remained warm and mobile she was safe. When you feel well enough to get out of bed and your body tells you the worst is over, you can gradually start building up your basic vitality again with good foods and natural vitamins and minerals—not too quickly, though, or those viruses will latch onto the strong new cells you're presenting to them. It is better to wait for a week or two before you start the rebuilding process, so that all the rubbish and dead viruses can be cleaned away before you start.

The way to avoid the flu is to stay warm, making sure you always take a coat no matter how fine and mild the weather is when you start off in the morning. Winter time is influenza time, the time when you are more likely to suffer sudden chills.

BRONCHITIS

Bronchitis is a convenient tag to hang on a disease we all know but perhaps do not know sufficiently well to combat its repeated attacks. Bronchitis—inflammation and infection of the bronchial system—can come from so many different causes, some of them obvious but many of them obscure. Do you know that you can get bronchitis because your kidneys are not functioning strongly enough? That you can also get bronchitis if your sinuses are under-performing, your tonsils are weak, or your mother-in-law is bugging you? Ill-health and disease are often the result of stress, and not necessarily stress in the bronchial tree. A lung weakened by physical trauma is obviously more susceptible to bronchial troubles than a strong, healthy lung. We all breathe in polluted air— it's a fact of life we can't escape, and only its degree is variable —so we all breathe in material irritant to lung tissues. But a healthy lung can handle anything that's thrown at it, just as the body as a whole can overcome stress of many kinds with remarkable ease if it is healthy. I always aim to restore to my patients a pair of strong lungs immune to any stress-causing or damage-causing irritant factors. I treat bronchitic people with a variety of herbs: coltsfoot, which heals and soothes irritated membranes; garlic, to deal with infection; grindelia, a specific herb for bronchial asthmatic conditions; liquorice, which we all know as that black, sticky stuff staining our children's tongues and keeping our bowels moving; comfrey to heal ragged, torn tissues and rebuild healthy ones in their place; and other herbs as indicated by the individual patient's total picture.

A simple home treatment to soothe inflammation and remove possible infection in bronchial conditions is my friend, and yours, garlic. Garlic holds the answer if the condition arises mainly from bacterial infection of the lungs and the bronchial tree. You could take up to twenty garlic capsules or about forty odourless garlic tablets per day without any harm whatsoever to your body—though they could induce diarrhoea and stomach discomfort if there is a lot of waste matter to remove. (But note that garlic is contra-indicated if you have liver or gall, pancreas or bile problems.) As well as the cleansing garlic treatment, you can give yourself inhalations of peppermint oil. Go to your health store for peppermint oil, put two drops in a basin, then pour on about a pint (600 millilitres) of boiling water. Steam yourself over the fumes, which will not only clear your head and bronchial tree but refresh and deodorise your whole household.

Peppermint oil has a penetrating and cleansing action, calming the bronchial nerves and loosening phlegm. People who suffer from this type of disease often have difficulty in sleeping well because their breathing is laboured and uncom-fortable. A simple remedy is to dab a few drops of peppermint oil on a paper tissue and tack it with a pin or drawing-pin somewhere about the head of the bed, being careful to keep it away from eyes and nostrils. Don't, whatever you do, put the tissue beside or underneath your pillow, or you may roll against it in the night and finish up with very sore eyes or burnt skin. This is a powerful and a volatile oil that will vaporise gradually during the night so that you breathe in its fumes over many hours. This simple treatment can be used in conjunction with the garlic, lemon and honey mixture for colds, to help your breathing during the night. You can also rub a little eucalyptus oil on the chest area, as our grand-mothers did, remembering again that this strong, pure oil can burn, and must be kept away from eyes, ears, lips and nostrils. The delightful Victorian custom of hanging a block of camphor round the neck in a little red flannel bag was really a forerunner of natural therapy. The vibrations of the colour red combined with the penetrating action of the slowly vaporising camphor to provide both a treatment and a preventive measure.

Castor oil, too, can be used for bronchitis—but for goodness' sake don't take the stuff internally. Smear the chest and bronchial areas liberally with warm castor oil (blood temperature only, and test it with your finger). Cover the whole area with an old piece of sheeting (or red flannel if you are a purist), then retire to bed in your oldest nightclothes. Castor oil penetrates into the skin and down to unhappy lungs, and will draw out all sorts of toxic material and waste matter. Whatever treatment you are taking internally can be boosted along with a castor-oil poultice.

The old mustard plaster is just as effective today as it was when Jill mended Jack's head with mustard, vinegar and brown paper. The mustard and vinegar are smeared on the *outside* of a piece of brown paper, which is then laid against the chest, ensuring that the skin is not burnt by the strength of the ingredients. Put a warm towel or blanket over this poultice and leave for half an hour to an hour; and keep the patient warm afterwards as well.

HIGH BLOOD PRESSURE

Victims of high blood pressure seem bent on self-destruction. Who in the engineering world would ask an air-conditioning system to work at all under twice its loading and half its efficiency levels, or expect rusted water-pipes clogged with flaking metal and corrosion to deliver a required pressure without breakdown? Yet many patients—some of them engineers—look at me with disbelief when I try to explain how stupid it is to try to force a large volume of fluid through a small, clogged aperture when it is so easy to rebore the canal. They say, 'I don't overload my heart, I don't do strenuous exercise. Just give me something to stop me feeling dizzy and so tired.' I can certainly do that if they insist, but by the time

I have finished talking to them they very seldom do. I tell them how many stress points they have in their circulatory system that could blow or seize up at any moment, and they sit there goggle-eyed, convinced that they are about to leave this world until I reassure them: they are not nearly dead but merely dumb! I explain how the health of the system can be restored and how their whole attitude to life will change for the better once the pressurised flow of blood and oxygen through the tubes is normalised: stamina will increase, there will be less fatigue, sex will become again the natural release it was meant to be. And now I have the patient's interest for whatever treatment is to follow.

Boiled onions are part of this treatment, as are all members of the onion family: leeks, shallots, chives, garlic, and the common onion, either brown or white. The onion and its relatives contain a unique principle that loosens, changes and releases lumps of cholesterol-loaded deposit along the internal walls of the heart and its arteries and veins. That's a basic simple treatment in itself; but a naturopath or herbalist like myself adds a herbal mixture containing several specific remedies for this condition, amongst which are stinging nettle and rue, together with whatever other herbs apply to the individual patient's condition. Lecithin has a similar action to that of the onion family, breaking up and removing choking cholesterol deposits from many body tissues. It is something everyone over the age of thirty odd, either with or without a family history of circulatory disease, can have daily as a dietary supplement, not only to remove any deposits lining the circulatory system but also to prevent such accumulations occurring in the first place.

ACHES AND PAINS

Luckily we don't all have major disease conditions like high blood pressure or bronchitis all of the time, and often the hardest to shift are the small everyday aches and pains that

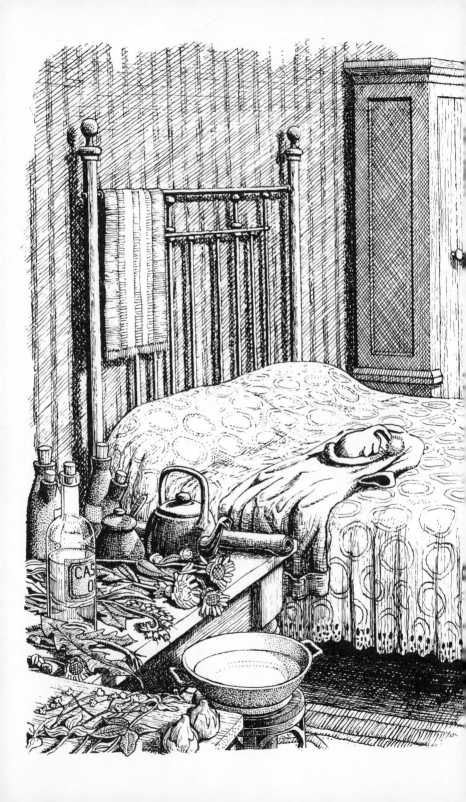

afflict us all from job stresses. No matter what muscle it is that is tight, hard and knotted, painful to touch and even more painful to use, there are several simple oils that you can rub into it to relax the taut muscle fibres and remove the pain and inflammation. Wintergreen oil is a good old-fashioned remedy for muscular aches and pains. It gives its strong characteristic odour to many proprietary lines used for rubbing liniments, for sports injury embrocations, and as an ingredient in salves and lotions to ease rheumatic or muscular pain. Its strong camphor-like odour is unmistakable, saturating the hands of the sports-medicine masseur and wafting out the windows of your friendly osteopath. The pure oil is highly concentrated and must be used broken down with a bland rubbing oil such as almond, safflower, or whichever vegetable oil suits your skin best. Don't use pure wintergreen oil undiluted on any skin surface whatsoever, for it can burn and redden, not only sensitive skin but skin in exposed areas of the body. It will penetrate up to 3 inches (7 or 8 centimetres) deep into tight muscles and aching bones. It is also specifically indicated for acute muscular conditions such as lumbago, sciatica, and fibrositis, unlocking muscles that have seized up tight against the bony skeleton, rendering that part of the body immobile. Wintergreen has been synthesised and made artificially under its chemical name of methylsalicilate, and this is the name it goes by in preparations on the pharmacist's shelf. You can feel almost instantaneously the powerful heat generated in the affected area when this oil is lightly massaged into the skin. The warmth lasts for hours, gently unlocking deep muscles and releasing their tight hold on the bones. If you don't mind smelling like a prize-fighter for a little while, get your husband or wife or a helpful member of your family to rub sore spots with wintergreen oil as soon as they appear, preventing secondary build-up of muscular tension.

Rosemary oil does a similar job, but it does it more gently, calming and relaxing the nerves and muscles at the same time. Rosemary oil is indicated for those headaches at the temples and behind the eyes after a stressful day in town or a long day's drive when eyes are screwed up against the glare along the road, or when concentration or study has tightened up the muscles around the forehead and eye area. Any headaches produced from muscular tension can be eased by rubbing a little pure rosemary oil, not diluted at all, gently into the area with the fingertips. If the headache is from a muscular cause it will be dispelled within minutes. Some migraine-type headaches can be eased with an application of rosemary oil to the back of the neck and high up into the cranial area; but a true migraine headache is a different problem altogether. When this type of headache originates from neck muscles clamping tight around vertebrae and cervical nerves, rub rosemary oil gently but firmly into the muscle area. Don't forget to add a couple of drops of the same rosemary oil to the rinsing water when washing your hair. It is not an oily oil, and will not make your hair look greasy and dull; it will strengthen, tone, and stimulate the hair roots and therefore the hair growth and condition. Keep a small bottle of rosemary oil in the medicine cupboard, for there is bound to be at least one member of your family who needs its soothing relief from time to time. Consult your naturopath or osteopath or chiropractor, or all three, to track down the source of any headache problem that refuses to respond to applications of rosemary oil.

HEADACHES AND MIGRAINE

Headaches come second on the list after the common cold as the most popular disease of humanity in general. It must have all happened when we began to hold our heads upright instead of dropping them on the ends of our necks as anthropologists tell us we did. The neck and its nerves and the branches rising therefrom into the head and face are vulnerable areas to muscular stress and therefore pain. Misplacement of the vertebrae in the neck and upper dorsal area can cause headache problems, but the tone of the muscles must also be considered, so that when your chiropractor has put the bones back where they belong, the muscles should then be conditioned and strengthened to keep them there.

Migraine headaches are the worst of all. Migraine people are like asthma people and ulcer people and indigestion people: they exhibit physically a reaction to stress. I have many migraine patients and they are all brave people who hide from the world their wrongs and their woes, keeping a stiff upper lip and acting as if they were in absolute control of their emotional and physical tensions. True migraines appear only after the originating stress has passed—the Friday night syndrome, you might call it. The person concerned battles on all the week, rising to the occasion, being unflappable no matter what, generally handling difficult situations—apparently without dropping his bundle. The bundle drops only when there is no further need to carry it. He may go for weeks or months carrying everybody else's strife and problems, then he may drop the whole lot in one blinding, crashing, flattening migraine headache.

During an attack a true migraine sufferer cannot stand glare or light, needs absolute quiet and rest in a darkened room, may vomit spasmodically for an hour or for twenty-four, and may pass through the headache stage to a state of absolute flatness and emptiness physically and mentally. The pattern may not be as bad as this, but mostly these general symptoms are found, together with a typical pattern along the outside rim of the iris of the eye, which tells an iridologist that here is a true migraine reaction to stress.

Natural treatment of this type of disease involves what any other type of natural treatment should involve: an assessment of the patient as a whole person, an individual totally different from any other individual, and exhibiting certain physical signs that represent the emotional and mental patterns of reaction to their own particular stresses. Migraine sufferers are often placid people on the surface, but tight physically with the resultant occlusion of the nerves of the upper neck resulting in their headaches. The treatment of migraine sufferers is a long and sometimes next-to-impossible task— that of getting them to relieve their tensions openly and outwardly so as to avoid the physical build-up that produces the headache. I would not advise you to treat your migraine headaches with any simple home remedy—other than kicking the cat or hurling a few old dinner plates at the wall to break the pattern of sitting tight and calm upon your problems. The natural treatment of a migraine sufferer is aimed at gently but firmly releasing stresses and tensions through natural channels, while physically undoing the tight nervous control system that also controls the muscles and the emotional reactions.

THE LIVER

How do you know whether your liver is healthy or not? There are some outwardly visible signs of an inward functional imbalance that are familiar to any of you who have wassailed rather heavily and woken the next morning with your liver decidedly unhappy. The eyes are bloodshot and perhaps even yellow, with dark circles beneath them, and the tissue tone of the body can only be described as 'sagging'. It's what you could call 'the morning after' feeling happening all the time. Dr Alfred Vogel, the Swiss doctor who has pioneered so many treatments in the field of natural health, has written a whole volume on the liver. He regards its efficient functioning as so important to the balanced state of the whole body that he devotes chapter after chapter to what you should do to keep your liver happy. I spent some time with him in Switzerland recently and his bounding health and superb vitality at the age of seventy-two convinced me that if your liver is happy, then you are happy too. He trotted me around Zurich faster than I had ever trotted along city streets before, talking incessantly of the joy and the vigour and the health he would wish for everyone on this earth. He took me to lunch at a delightful health-food restaurant, talking to and exhorting many of its patrons to eat whatever would keep the liver happy. 'Carrots!' He threw his hands up in the air and gesticulated as he spoke to anyone who wanted to listen on the glories of the carrot, the virtues of the dandelion, the mountain mosses he had found so effective in liver complaints, the mineral water on the tables for the patrons, the natural vegetable oils cold-pressed from their seeds or kernels, which supply the liver with its fatty acids; he progressed from table to table leaving devoted liver-lovers behind him!

The liver performs so many complex functions that its health can almost be said to denote the health level of the whole body. It is the chemical factory changing processed foodstuffs presented to it by the stomach into biologically useful compounds available to body tissues. How do you know when your liver is not happy? You will know, all right; but if you wish to confirm the fact, you can dig in all four fingers of your right hand under your right rib-cage as deeply as you can, and if you feel even vague discomfort your liver is not as good as it should be. If you are so overweight that you can't even get your fingers in underneath your ribs it goes without saying that your liver is overloaded. What do you do to get it back to normal functioning again? First of all, you eat dandelions, and you drink dandelions, and if it's bad enough you consult your naturopathic physician and he or she prescribes dandelion for you in medicinal-sized quantities. Dandelion coffee is one of the best things that ever happened to a doubtful liver. It is made from the roasted roots of the dandelion and nothing else, and on its own it can provide a tonic lift for a sad liver and make it a happy liver once again.

If you drink a great deal of black coffee or a great deal of alcohol, or both, you are a subject for liver problems. Caffeine, found in great quantities in black coffee, is like dealing your liver a karate chop every time you drink it; and the same picture applies to alcohol, particularly spirits. Coffee and alcohol may keep your body going when it feels terribly tired and is begging for rest and recuperation time; but the liver is going to have to take the brunt of the strain. If you have had hepatitis or any weakening liver disease, dandelion coffee on its own can be a simple home remedy to renew the full function of the liver without any other treatment whatsoever. It can provide this vital organ with the correct natural balance of everything it needs to restore peak function.

Feeling a bit liverish right now? I'd not be surprised, for the liver is rather strangely connected to the emotional centres, and even talking about it can build up stress that can be felt by a liver doubtful of its own performance. Some ancient philosophers believed the liver, not the heart or the nervous system, to be the seat of the emotions, and it is certainly true that an inefficiently functioning liver can produce many symptoms of mental or emotional illness. There are many complicated treatments for a liver that is structurally or chemically inefficient, but the everyday weed, dandelion, can rebalance and rebuild until normal function is restored.

ALLERGIES

Allergies are becoming more and more common in civilised populations. An allergy is not a disease state in itself but only a symptom of an erratically functioning immune system, where anything from a mosquito bite to a strawberry can be interpreted as a violently dangerous intrusion; and the puffed-up eyes and running nose, or the violently itchy blistery rash over the entire body, calls for a shot of adrenalin or heavy cortisone therapy from a medical practitioner as a last-ditch attempt to help your body overcome its frantic distress. You all know someone who has allergy reactions in springtime, or allergy reactions to house-dust, or prawns or cats—or even to people, so that having a particular person around may bring on a fit of the sneezes.

Allergy reaction tests merely tell you which triggering

substances to stay away from. They don't tell you *why* you are allergic, and the reason why is the concern of natural therapy. What is important is not what substances you are allergic to, but the fact that you have a disordered immune reaction: it is this that needs treatment. Your body is telling you that these substances are hurting it, and the reason for this can be dealt with by several simple measures.

If a person is allergic to cat's hair, we say, 'So what? How this came about is secondary to the fact that the mucous membranes of that person are irritated by some substance in an unnatural manner.' Any agent that can be inhaled into the breathing passages or up into the nasal and sinus areas comes under one class of allergic reaction, and these are best dealt with by strengthening the mucous linings to a state of natural health and resilience, so that they will no longer be irritated by a substance that should not normally be harmful to humans. Mucous linings are hyper-sensitised in allergic subjects, and we must try to desensitise them to arrest distress signals that rush out into the bloodstream and the metabolic pattern each time the substance is inhaled.

One of the simplest treatments as a dietary corrective measure is to eat bananas. Don't throw up your hands and say they will make you fat: they won't. All you need is one or two bananas per day, more if you enjoy them. Sounds too simple? The reasons why are biologically complex, but basically the virtue of bananas lies in a combination of a bland protein with vitamin A and D balance and a trace of bromine and the correct balance of iron with other elements, together with many other interrelated factors that can make the banana almost a perfect food item for sufferers from allergic reactions.

We are only speaking here of foods and substances that are not in themselves dangerous to human health. It's a vastly different story if a person is working with harmful chemicals, with photographic solutions, with hairdressing preparations, with industrial dusts or acid solutions, or any of the other substances that the body is quite justified in rejecting as potentially or actually harmful. The treatment of the patient in these circumstances means deciding whether he or she can continue at that occupation knowing that health is breaking down—as well as taking a diet containing bananas while making the decision to stay or go.

Bloodstream allergies are somewhat different, for the body is reacting to a substance that is either in contact with the skin and absorbed through it into the bloodstream, or has pierced through the skin like a mosquito-bite or a wasp-sting, a tick-bite or a nettle sting. You all know the irritative qualities of such a sting that, with scratching, can become a reddened area covered in weeping blisters before a day has elapsed; and this area can grow until the body can get into a state of anaphylactic shock in extreme cases. A simple home treatment is to drink alfalfa tea or take alfalfa tablets to correct this allergic pattern by counterbalancing the excessive acids of the protein poison with a heavily alkaline-producing agent. Alfalfa's correct proportions of all amino acids in a vegetable form help your body to neutralise the introduced protein agent.

Allergy reactions can be lumped together and called a new defence system over-developed by the body to give warning signs when metabolic processes cannot handle a substance in a normal manner. The dramatic increase in allergic asthma, in skin allergies, in sinus over-production of mucus, have all happened as our environment becomes more and more loaded down with artificially introduced substances. Natural living in a simple fashion tends to produce vast improvement for an allergy sufferer. Bodies are becoming 'afraid', and they fight off outside agents with such ferocity that a violent allergy is often the consequence.

Sufferers from these symptoms can also revert to another old-fashioned natural food supplement—cod-liver oil. Taken as prescribed, this can naturally rebuild the body's mucous linings to a better state of health, so that they can repel apparently dangerous or genuinely dangerous agents. A vitamin B source of foodstuffs, such as wheatgerm or yeast or liver, can also help allergy sufferers by strengthening their nervous systems, which can become overloaded by all this sensory distress.

My intention here is to give you an outline in a simple fashion of how you can help yourself at home by using simple corrective dietary and health procedures to achieve a better state of vital health. All manner of illnesses could be discussed, and the same principle would apply: the aim of natural treatment is always to strengthen the structure, the function, and the vitality of the part of the body concerned in the illness, and not necessarily to relieve the symptoms, which will disappear of their own accord when the basic reason for the ill-health is removed. If you have diseases stemming from an imbalance in the digestion, then step up the calcium levels and the other appropriate vitamins and minerals by way of herbs and natural simple foods so that the alimentary tract is better able to handle whatever food is presented to it. If you suffer from a disease of the nervous system—headaches and tension problems, a hypertensive condition, a pathological condition of the physical nerves—then the obvious treatment is to strengthen the nervous system by providing a better balance of the substances it needs to function correctly, the vitamin B and phosphorus and magnesium from natural sources.

A living human being is an incredibly complex combination of moving parts motivated by chemically instructed processes; and it is so designed that, given the simple conditions of rest and exercise, of growth of new cells and destruction of old, of the correct kinds of fuel in food and drink, and a balance in the emotional climate, it can protect itself from actual or potential disease conditions. No one ever heals anybody: if a practitioner knows his business and uses his knowledge and understanding, he can only provide the conditions for a body to set about healing itself. The longer I work with the human body and the personalities of the people that live in it, the more respect I have for the Creator.

If you are healthy, you don't get sick! Natural methods concentrate on health rather than disease; and it never fails to astonish me that such thinking can be branded as quackery. How logical it is to aim at strengthening or normalising all the functional and structural parts of the body, at sorting out the emotional problems too; how logical to aim at rebalancing the body as a whole!

8

What is Health?

Anyone who feels healthy feels happy. That's a broad statement, but I've never yet found it proved wrong. You may say that the opposite will necessarily follow, that anyone who is happy is healthy, and in most cases this is so. But I have known patients with serious illnesses who have impressed me as being 'healthy' people.

One I shall never forget. Her husband had to carry her, stiff and deformed with advanced rheumatoid arthritis, like a little grotesque wooden doll, up the few steps at my door. Her hands were clawed and emaciated like hawk's talons, her feet clubbed and hunched into special shoes; she had two plastic knee joints and two plastic hip joints and in the middle of these four serious operations some enthusiastic surgeon had performed a total hysterectomy. The arthritis had set her neck in a vice and had even crept into her jawbone, but I have never seen such a radiant, real smile and such blue unclouded eyes. We talked about her problems, and her calmness and peace astounded me.

'Are you a strongly religious person?' I asked her.

'No,' she said, smiling gently.

'Then where do you find the strength to be so happy'— I gestured at her body, cramped and twisted in the chair— 'in amongst all this?'

She answered me with another smile, 'I made up my mind over seventeen years ago, when I first realised how my illness would progress, that it would affect no one else but me. It was *my* illness and I would not impose it on my husband, family or friends. I'm happier this way.'

To me, that woman was in a state of health. I could help her with herbs to alleviate and soothe her condition, but to undo the structural damage to her body was impossible and she had come not to ask me for miracles, only for a little more strength. Whenever a patient sits by my desk complaining that his or her lot is much worse than anyone else's I try to think of that other patient and her contented smile.

Physical perfection, the Mr Universe type of health, seems to me to be only a partial substitute for the real thing. The fitness fanatic who beats his hairy chest, claiming that if we all ran miles each morning, drank nothing but apple juice, and ate only raw foods with our shining, regularly spaced teeth, we should all be as happy as he is, is fooling his audience as well as himself. Complete absorption in one's own health is, I believe, a form of chronic illness. Think of the time and energy that individual spends selfishly! 'How can I get rid of the wrinkles around my eyes, the bulge under my waistband?' 'Is my weight up a few grams this morning?' 'Is my tongue furry, white, yellow, cracked or sore?' 'There are several hairs that came out on the comb; am I going bald?' 'When I'm forty I must not look a day over twenty-five.'

I know people like this who make their own life and the lives of everyone around them a continuing series of small miseries and large apprehensions. The frown lines increase with every calorie they count and with every new diet they follow. They become more disillusioned when the promised health and beauty refuse to materialise.

My purpose has been to show you how to promote physical health and well-being, but *not* to make you obsessed with this aim. As with every other natural process, balance is the state to achieve. My little arthritic patient endured physical pain and deformity to balance her beautiful, calm soul; the fashion model with proud head and slim neck is stricken with crippling migraines; the teetotal vegetarian can get gout from a calcium deficiency just as surely as he can mock at his sozzled fellow-sufferer for drinking too much port and eating lobster mornay twice a week.

The health answer seems to be a sensible blend of what is good for the body, the mind, and even the soul. It consists not of self-mastery but of a certain amount of self-forgetting. If you have a pain here today and there tomorrow and the next day not at all, that's OK—it's over and done with. If you have a twinge of sciatica one day, then persistently for a week or a month, it would be a sensible idea to do something about it, not endure it uncorrected. But if you put up with recurring asthma attacks for twenty years, becoming a pathetic martyr to a set of symptoms that can be corrected by natural commonsense treatment of the cause of the distress, then good health is not for you because you don't care enough about it.

I had an eighty-three-year-old patient some months ago who had the healthiest constitution I have ever encountered. His body was lithe and in good muscular condition; his eyes were like those of a kitten, clear, wide, and a brilliant blue; his voice was firm and he spoke with the self-confidence of a man who has lived his life according to a strong but gentle philosophy. He had hurt his shoulder chopping firewood, had had cortisone therapy from a doctor, and had subsequently broken out in an irritable rash on his legs, arms and chest.

He came to me in a state of puzzlement. 'I have never been sick,' he said, 'never. This is awful. Why do people put up with illness?' He had been a timber-worker all his life, raised a sturdy family, and enjoyed every facet of living. He was surprised and hurt, like a child who has been punished unjustly. 'We were never meant to be sick,' he said in a disgusted tone as I prescribed herbs for him. He was dead right. The natural state of animal and man is health. An animal knows instinctively what to eat, how to rest or fast altogether to correct an unnatural state of illness. Man thinks too much about it, perhaps. When instinct tells you to stay in bed and drink fruit juice during a heavy cold, but economic necessity goads you into getting up and going to the office to eat a heavy business lunch with an important client, the body will complain to the extent of becoming overloaded and really ill, perhaps even chronically ill. Here is where the ulcers start and the blood pressure soars and the tension headaches begin, ensuring that the physical circuits are always overloaded and under stress.

One of my first questions to a new patient is always 'What's your occupation?' My next question is always 'Do you still want to be an accountant?' (or typist, clerk, dancer, musician or whatever it is). He sometimes replies, 'No, I hate it, but I have to keep it up.' Then I sit there being difficult and say, 'Why?' I get a variety of answers, none of which convinces the patient or me. If your job stress is enough to cause persistent chronic illness, then either you break the stress pattern by a conscious effort at habit-changing or you switch jobs. It sounds simple again, and it *is* simple.

The typist with a chronic pain in her right shoulder and right side of her neck must be treated for her symptoms, yes, but also for the cause of those symptoms, the fact that she constantly turns her head and upper body to the left to scan her copy. She does this under stress conditions, with an impatient boss breathing sometimes literally down her neck;

her right-neck and shoulder muscles tense and lock against the strain, and pain, inflammation, and loss of mobility result. It's so simple to change her shorthand notes to the right-hand side, to sit in the bus going home looking out the window on the right-hand side, to move her favourite TV chair to the opposite side of the room, deliberately breaking the pattern that caused the problem. She is consciously removing many of the causes of the stress. But if it's really her boss who is her main problem, the tension will not wholly disappear until she gets herself a new job with a different boss.

A man who loves outdoor work perhaps has chronic chest or bronchial troubles. He must first be treated with natural medicines and diet and rest; but he must also be faced with the question, 'Why then are you working in an air-conditioned office, with a rotten awful draught blowing straight at your nose, throat and chest from a vent situated in the wrong spot in relation to your desk?' Fear of financial loss or a drop in job status or plain fear of a plunge into the unknown may inhibit the intense desire of a patient to change his occupation. When this happens a pattern of chronic, severe, almost untreatable, illness may appear: And here are the ulcer victims, the executives with excruciatingly painful migraine headaches every Friday night, the people with strokes, high blood pressure, digestive troubles, who end up as pill-poppers whose day is divided into small time-slots between medications.

I have several patients from major companies that give periodic cholesterol-level checks to their top executives. Key men are hard to find, expensive to train, and a major company asset, so their continuing health is a matter of prime importance to the balance sheet. I get a frantic phone call saying, 'Our check-up is coming at the end of the month. Help!' I have told of simple procedures to follow for reducing cholesterol levels and breaking up existing cholesterol deposits; and these men go on a crash programme of boiled onions, garlic—the whole works. None of them has ever failed to pass his cholesterol check-up, and none of them has ever listened to my advice to change jobs.

One completely happy professional man did listen. He was a dentist, with so many sites of illness, pain, weakness and general debility all over his body that I filled up his complete case-card like a map of the world. He had aches and pains, infections and inflammations, wind, hay fever, stomach ulcers and—worst of all—ingrown toe-nails. After many appointments he came to the same conclusion as I did—he not only did not want to be a dentist now, but had never wanted to be a dentist. He went straight out from the last appointment I ever had with him, put his practice on the market, and bought a cement truck. When I last saw him, he and his wife and family were leaving in a caravan for a tour round Australia for twelve months or more on the money he had made from his cement truck. I have never heard mention of another ache or pain in any of the letters I have had from him or his wife from different parts of the country. When he gets his rebellion out of his system, he may even go back to dentistry and still not have an ache or a pain.

One of the main causes of physical ill-health stems from early conditioning of a child or teenager or young adult into a pattern that is not the right pattern for him. The proud father with an intelligent, mathematically minded son wants him to carry on the family business of engineering: he may be forcing that son into ill-health both physical and mental. I have had so many patients confessing, 'I never really wanted to...' And what they 'never really wanted to' is what they have been doing most of their lives to please somebody else or to gain affection or security or peace. Many of them decide to continue this pattern, knowing that it is someone else's pattern and not their own. And this is the cause of the continuing stress condition we have found to be one of the main causes of chronic illness.

Let me quote to you from Emerson a paragraph that embodies my thoughts on health. 'The first wealth is health. Sickness is poor spirited, and cannot serve anyone; it must husband its resources to live. But health answers its own ends and has to spare; runs over, and inundates the neighbourhoods and creeks of other men's necessities.' Rabelais had some untypical thoughts on health too: 'Without health life is not life; it is only a state of languor and suffering—an image of death.' What a waste!

There are so many things to do, to enjoy, to give, to take, to learn—what a waste of time and life being sick! The saddest patients of all are the ones who steadfastly refuse to get better. They need to be sick. These are the ones who have given up the struggle and retreated into illness as an excuse. Hard words, perhaps, but true. The body is such a vital self-renewing organism that there are few illnesses it cannot repair and throw off given natural treatment, time, rest and common sense. 'Joy, temperance, and repose, slam the door on the doctor's nose.' Longfellow must have been a practising naturopath!

Let me wish you the strength, the vitality, the joy and contentment that a balanced state of good health can give you.

Index

When necessary, main page numbers are distinguished by the use of bold type.